MW01243669

At Home with
Dementia

Insightful Caregiver Strategies for Smarter Decisions, Safer Outcomes and Improved Sanity

Reginald A. Lawson

Copyright © 2020 by Reginald A. Lawson

At Home with Dementia: *Insightful Caregiver Strategies for Smarter Decisions, Safer Outcomes and Improved Sanity*
by Reginald A. Lawson

All rights reserved. No part of this publication may be reproduced, stored in a retrieval system or transmitted in any way by any means, electronic, mechanical, photocopy, recording or otherwise without the written permission of the author. Reviewer may quote brief passages in reviews.

While all attempts have been made to verify the information provided in this publication, neither the author nor the publisher assumes any responsibility for errors, omissions, or contrary interpretation of the subject matter herein.

The views expressed in this publication are those of the author alone and should not be taken as expert instructions or commands. The reader is responsible for his or her own actions, as well as his or her own interpretation of the material found within this publication.

Adherence to all applicable laws and regulations, including international, federal, state and local governing professional licensing, business practices, advertising, and all other aspects of doing business in the US, Canada or any other jurisdiction is the sole responsibility of the reader and consumer.

Neither the author nor the publisher assumes any responsibility or liability whatsoever on behalf of the consumer or reader of this material. And received slight of any individual or organization is purely unintentional.

Book design by Reginald A. Lawson   Cover design by Vanessa Mendozzi
ISBN: 978-1-7344772-2-1

DEDICATION

This book is dedicated to the life and memory of an angelic warrior, my mother:

Gloria Natalie Lawson Gross Black

Reginald A. Lawson

TABLE OF CONTENTS

FOREWORD

Reginald has given us much more than a book. This is a tool! He gets the point, and helps you resolve the realities of what to do and how to do it.

My caregiving journey started while I was serving as County Executive. Saying I had a full plate is an understatement. I appreciate, as a Caregiver, the need for a clear vision of what I am facing, and this provides that.

The shared lessons from Reginald's journey will help new and veteran Caregivers navigate the often-changing moments associated with cognitive illness care, in particular, and all caregiving in general.

He provides insightful solutions at a level all Caregivers can understand to enhance their knowledge and confidence.

This Caregiver GPS tool is one of the best reference guides for whatever part of the journey you are on. It refreshingly highlights the honorable and positive moments embedded in the giving. This is the book I wish I had in the beginning. It will be my co-pilot throughout the remainder of my journey.

The Honorable Rushern L. Baker III
Caregiver & Former County Executive,
Prince George's County, Maryland

FASTEN YOUR CAREGIVER'S SEATBELT

As soon as the doctor said, "Your mother has dementia" I thought, "Now what?"

There were three truths I started this dementia journey with: 1) I made a commitment to do all I could to not institutionalize my mother; 2) I had no idea what dementia was; and 3) I had no idea what at-home caregiving would require. ***Now I do!***

Let's be really clear, dementia is an unrelenting, multifaceted condition unlike any other. Its diverse types and stages, mixed with a person's personality, creates unique scenarios. My initial research provided clinical perspectives about dementia and its challenges. Those understandings were not even close to what I would need to provide care and preserve my sanity.

At Home with Dementia is for all who want an up-close view of what to expect on this journey and are searching for additional approaches to help care for their loved one.

The requirements for nursing home dementia care can be devastating emotionally, physically and financially. Often times care at home is your only option.

This book is about **the challenges, the humility, the honor, and the goodness** involved with being a dementia caregiver.

At-home caregivers need to learn insightful, effective and efficient strategies and tactics to address the sufferer's childlike behavior, attitudes, and forgetfulness while keeping them safe and respecting their adulthood.

My dementia caregiving challenges were multidimensional. I lived two hours away, worked during the day, coached during the evenings and weekends and rarely slept more than five hours on any given day.

You, like myself, may have family and friends who care and pray, but are physically or emotionally unavailable to consistently help. Prayer does help; however, you will need reliable, proven approaches as a dynamic GPS for this journey.

My scenarios and suggestions are real life, not fictional or studied in a lab. I continue to speak with countless people about their dementia caregiving journey. When we talk, we are inevitably surprised and uplifted—and sometimes saddened—by common and often identical scenarios we share. We recognized each other and our loved ones in our experiences.

It took me four scary and often painful years to understand, refine and validate the insights herein. Apply these insights for yourself and your loved one. You will learn about the roles and realities of being a caregiver, as well as the need for a POA, Trustee and all around go-to person.

At Home with Dementia is divided into four sections to educate you on how to:

- develop an enlightened caregiver's mindset for gaining, improving and maintaining your sanity (Saner),

- gain insights to reduce fears of inadequacy and to improve understandings and decision making (Smarter),

- identify and defeat dementia-enabling threats in, around and outside the home (Safer), and,

- develop a strategic checklist of who and what are useful, and when to implement tactics. (Scenarios)

Lastly, this book is my attempt to provide a reality check, a buffer for your sanity—which will definitely be tested. The goal is to provide refreshing perspectives to help you appreciate that aspects of caregiving are a privilege and an honor, despite its frustrations and struggles. Apply these insights to help make wiser informed decisions, have safer outcomes and experience improved sanity.

Reginald A. Lawson

HER INDOMITABLE SPIRIT

When "D" stood for dynamic and determined.

This dementia journey was just a segment of my mother's lifespan. Gloria Natalie Lawson, born May 14, 1938, in Valdosta, GA, was a "Scrapper in life". She had the grit of a warrior and the heart of an angel.

My mother 's Valdosta home had dirt floors and a freight train railroad track just thirty feet from the front door. The family migrated to Wilmington, DE, from 1945 to 1950. Her initial Wilmington home was a small second level, two-bedroom apartment with wooden floors, ceiling lights and paved streets outside. The North was different and faster paced. She grew up contending with the daily prejudice thrown at a southerner in the South and the North. She was told to know her place and don't speak unless spoken too. This indoctrination can cause a person to not ask for needed help, however, that was not the case for my mother.

My five feet one inch, about one-hundred twenty-five pounds, strong willed mother was inquisitive and tough as nails. She was excited with life insisting on knowing how and why things worked. My mother kept her home in an orderly manner. She knew exactly where things were in each closet and cabinet. Oh, you should not make the mistake of putting something in a place she did not have it initially. "Put things back exactly where you got it, or don't move it at all" she was known to say to anyone.

She was also particular about cleanliness. Maybe it was from her childhood or having to clean bedpans while working in the Veteran Administration Hospital as a nurse's aide.

She was a sharp dresser at all times. My mom grew up knowing how to wash and iron clothes. Her mother would have them ironing bedsheets. What I remembered, and admired, was how she would iron all twelve pairs of her work jeans, and her husband's jeans also. Those creases were sharp.

One of the things I truly cherished about my mom was her honesty and simplicity. She would tell you when she would or would not do something, and that was it. I am thankful for the gift of my mother. I gave her a Mother's Day card and a Father's Day card, for thirty-five consecutive years. She was that good and deserving. I had to do what I could to help her on this dementia journey. We had been through tough things before and I was confident this dementia thing was manageable. **Then I started seeing some of the signs of what was coming, of what dementia was doing to her:**

- Dressing sharply changed to dressing abstractly.

- She became reluctant to ask for or receive help.

- Her toughness turned into vulnerability and dependency.

- Things put into appropriate places moved to illogical places.

- Having a thought, became more and more, being loss-in-thought.

Some of the caregiving challenges associated with loved ones suffering cognitive illness can be daunting. Equally, some of the caregiving experiences can be rewarding in unforeseen ways. Read on to discover how to connect with, enjoy and reassure your loved-one as they journey into and out of dementia's evolving and consuming grip.

BECOMING SANER

Reginald A. Lawson

YOU'LL NEED MUCH MORE THAN CONFIDENCE FOR THIS JOURNEY

Caregiving will teach you new perspectives about yourself.

In most cultures, I suspect, it is a usual expectation for a parent to care for their child. They would stay up all hours of the night to calm fears and sickness. They ignore their own needs to meet their child's needs for protection and love.

Parents are the givers of care, children are the recipients of care, and the mission of child rearing is to prepare the child to leave the nest and live their own lives, dedicating themselves to meeting their own needs. I wager that it is less common to find an adult child who fully reciprocates that level of selfless care taking for their parent, at least in Western cultures.

I spent a minimum of one hour with my mother when I visited, no matter the purpose of the visit. Sometimes that was all I could reasonably spend. It took me approximately two hours, depending on the weather, State Troopers, time-of-day, and or traffic, to drive from my home in Maryland to hers in Delaware. Therefore, my visits needed a little more thought and planning as it was not efficient (meaning a good use of time and money) to turn around to gather a forgotten item.

I know what you are wondering. Yes, there were family members located much closer to my mother. Hold that thought until you read "Managing The Pains of Doubt."

I needed to be equally efficient in meeting my requirements as a professional consultant, since I would spend a minimum of four hours driving the car. The typical day spent visiting my mom would have me leaving at 6 in the morning and returning 11 at night. Many times, I had to deal with unanticipated issues during the commute and during visits. I often was so tired I did not remember several of my two-hour drives home at 1 a.m.

I recall on one occasion; I was in route to take my mother to a doctor's appointment. I always called her the day before, an hour prior to my leaving and about an hour prior to my arrival to remind her. She called me, during one of my commute to her, to insist I not waste my gas, as she had decided not to go to the doctor's office. I tried to change her mind, but she was having none of that. A part of me was thankful for the suggestion to not make the drive. My spirit overruled my logic telling me to stay the course. In retrospect, those occasions when she tried to talk me out of making the trip were some of the most important hours in our fading life together.

I saw her thankfulness and pride each time I walked through her door and her smile seemed sweeter. I could see the sense of order and thoughtfulness still alive in her demeanor when the dementia would give way. Many of those shared hours were not a test, but more of a testament.

A few things happened during each visit. My thinking changed, my values were enhanced, and my love deepened. My mother knew she had at least one person in this world she could count on. That mattered a whole lot to both of us. I would soon be looking around to see who or what I could count on, because the journey was getting bumpy.

Insight #1: *It's fine to be confident. It is wiser to first learn what to do and how to do it, and then build your confidence based on real outcomes.*

A MENTAL TUNEUP FOR THE JOURNEY

Denial does not make dementia easier. Build a mindset to overcome doubt, deceit, and attacks.

This section discusses challenges to my sense of correctness and order, expectations, doubts, and fears and strength to honor a promise to keep my mother in her home. Having dementia was my mother's greatest and scariest need. I constantly had this mindset that said, "This is on my watch and I can't fail." I now know the toll it took on **my wellness**.

I came to think of dementia as a living organism with a variable lifespan. I tried and tried to find things that would give me clear, valid indicators of which stage of dementia I was dealing with. I was most likely doing this because that approach works well for me in my professional and personal life, one in which I use logic and reasoning to assess each circumstance and possible outcomes.

Dementia was not cooperating with that approach. My insistence only revealed my inability to extend grace to myself, or to give peace-of-mind to my mother. I stubbornly asked doctors, nurses, other caregivers and hospice workers for definite signs and symptoms to look for, and specific meanings for what those signs meant or foretold. No one could or would say.

My conversations with caregivers (primary caregiver and family members) revealed that one of the things that makes living with dementia so darned hard is our degree of denial about the reality of the situation. We expect our loved one to reach a state of little or no growth or decline.

What actually happens with dementia is that there is often no "intermittent slowing or stopping." There is no point at which you (or even the doctors) can say with certainty that things will get no worse. The only certainty is the condition is unpredictable.

Decisions needed to be made, as with most things in life. There was no shortage of opinions of what could or should be done. However, you will find that dementia is not like most things. I hope the following becomes clear as you read these pages— **dementia is an attack on the quality of the sufferer's and caregiver's mental and physical life.**

You probably will go through these classic five stages of grief and loss:

1. Denial and Isolation

2. Anger

3. Bargaining

4. Depression

5. Acceptance

You could go back and forth in these stages with each new discovery on the journey. **Warning.** You will be accused, deceived, attacked, embarrassed and blamed. You will feel unappreciated and unwanted at times. *Don't let it stop you.*

I had to change my impeding way of thinking. Learn rightly that you will, as a caregiver, need to evolve emotionally, intellectually and spiritually with dementia. This is made more difficult, ironically, by the fact that your loved one's behavior and character will gradually become unrecognizable to you.

It took a while to develop and fine tune the successful outcomes that allowed her to stay in her comfortable and familiar home safely. I learned to look at new behavior with a *"Now what's she doing"* attitude. This way, I did not burden myself with self-induced frustration, anger or worry.

You, the caregiver, must take care of you—and that starts with adopting and applying a sanity-based mindset. Take advantage of my lessons to help you learn how to add dimensions to your heart and mind to reach the end of the journey with your sanity still vibrant.

Insight #2: *Always start with your mind set in input mode when connecting, in person or by video or phone, with your loved one. I found it helpful to expect change and treat it as the next thing to understand, to adapt to, and to overcome.*

MANAGING THE PAINS OF DOUBT

It can get lonely on this journey.

Dealing with dementia can hurt. The hurt will come from all kinds of sources. It will reveal things to you: your ignorance and weakness, your loved one's troubling traits and personality changes, the lack of assistance from family, friends, and neighbors.

You will be hurt from frustration with the greed of the medical industry, confusing and unhelpful laws, and unrelenting social norms that suggest people with cognitive issues should be put away at first sign of abnormality. The pain can happen each time you encounter a dementia-driven moment robbing you and your loved one of old normalcies. It hurts when they accuse you of stealing from them or wanting to harm them.

It hurts when you call out to family to share the load, if for only an hour, and nobody answers the call. It really hurts hearing, "You don't care about me! Get out of my house." However, the worst hurt comes from within yourself. It hurts when your frames of reference, experiences and common sense fail to yield an easy solution.

You may doubt your ability to manage the needed support. You may question your decision to try and provide direct care as opposed to institutionalizing your loved one. This gets really hard when your significant other, family, friends and well-wishers (but woefully informed) say things like, "I hate to see you wearing yourself out. Just put your mom in a nursing home and visit."

Pain can also reveal strength. I train my athletes to not focus so much on the part that is sore, but on the rest of the body that is working just fine. You will find you are more powerful, loving, resourceful, determined, trustworthy and compassionate than you realize. It helps to have an army of support, but it is not required. Being flexible and resourceful is what works best.

Understand this—If it falls to you to get it done, then you are most likely the better one for the journey. I believe there are people who are blessed with a spirit or ability to absorb the ills (body, mind, societal) of this world and allows them to function at a level above others.

Throughout this journey, and especially at the end, you may doubt yours, or others, decisions and actions. People occasionally would say, "You mean you are going to drive two hours up, stay two hours and then drive two hours back? Seems like a lot of time, money and gas. Would it not be easier to have someone else handle it?"

I had a math teacher that wanted to see your work so he could determine if you followed his method for arriving at your answer. Let others debate on the method, you just focus on getting the right answers for your circumstances. I had to, for the preservation of my sanity, categorize people's helpfulness. Some people, based on the situations, were supportive, indifferent, emotionally unavailable, or in the way. It was *easy* to determine a person's grouping. Ask for help with visiting, meals, bathing, doctor's or hair stylist appointments, food shopping or outings to the mall. **Real easy.**

I learned many things about human potential while serving as an athletic coach. All of us have limits. There are the mental limits (intelligence), emotional limits (willingness), and physical limits (movement). The most significant of these is our willingness—emotional capacity—to do something. Learn that there are unmeasurably good things that happen when you make an effort, a call, give a smile, or a hug. The value of your effort (result) is exponentially higher compared to the cost (method) involved.

Insight #3: *Modify your expectations to reduce your pain.*

Insight #4: *Don't beat people up if they can't handle things like you can. They usually mean well. Be thankful for your gift of how you persevere.*

Reginald A. Lawson

GETTING YOUR DEMENTIA LEARNER'S PERMIT

Learning how to hold on when dementia takes the wheel.

I get the cutest call from my well-organized mother. She asked, "Can you go with me next week so I can get this darn physical thing out of the way? You understand what they are talking about and can explain things better." I replied, "Absolutely I can!" I called the day before to remind her that I would pick her up around 8 am to go to the doctor, and she said, "OK, I'll be ready, see you then." I arrived at 8 am and she said, "Hey, what are you doing here?"

I responded, "To take you to see your doctor for your physical." She replied, "I don't have an appointment today." I pointed out that it was on her calendar. She said, "Well, you should have called me because I am not ready." I just smiled.

We, the caregivers, often tell outsiders how difficult the person suffering with dementia can be, sometimes all day long. Then all of a sudden, the sufferer starts to smile and act like everything is wonderful.[1]

Here we go: I am not making these things up. **These situations actually happened.** They served as milestones to adjust my thinking about what constitutes reasonable behavior on this journey. You should look for these signs.

And The Oscar Goes To. This happened between dementia stages one and two. My mother and I loved movies and would try to attend together a few times a year. This was our time. She was excited since it had been awhile since our last outing. We preferred going when the attendance was small. We got our warm buttered popcorn, candy and soda. Great seats in the center area. We even giggled like kids. "Quiet" she said as the lights dimmed.

About thirty minutes into the show, after the plot was revealed and main characters introduced, my mom gets up and goes out. I'm guessing it was for a bathroom run. Fifteen minutes later I go to see if she is OK. I have been known to knock on the door if I cannot find a lady to inquire for me.

No need to ask or knock this time. There was my mother leaning against the hallway wall. I asked her what was wrong. She said, "Nothing's wrong, I'm ready to go!" I had no idea what was going on. However, I knew that look and tone. I respectfully and immediately left the theater, abandoning the movie and all that good junk food. I believed this was the duality of dementia causing a short attention span and my mother's usual tone for telling you her decision about something.

The Cats. My mother disliked cats. There was a host of cats that often crossed her backyard. She decided to take her broom and chase a couple cats down the alley. Well, when she returned to the yard, she saw a cat trying to hide under the porch. She started banging against the lattice and broke it. The cat was gone, a new repair bill on the way.

Driving Me Crazy. My cousin was living with my mother and understood my mother should not drive. Well, my cousin wanted to get somethings from a few stores. I got calls from the neighbors that my mother was driving, with my cousin in the passenger seat each time. I asked my cousin if she lost her mind or wanted to lose her life. She said, "Your mom won't let me drive and said she would take me." At that point I learned I could not trust the two of them when it came to driving mom's car.

Peace-of-Mind at a Price. I informed my mother that she could not drive because the doctor felt it was unsafe and requested a medical suspension of driving privileges. My mother gave me this "Are you stupid" look and said, "I do what I want to do." I think it was more her determination to do what she wanted, then her dementia. (It can be difficult to understand, but some of your loved one's personality traits remain, and can become more entrenched, as dementia tightens its grip.)

Now I have to protect her from stubbornness (and her fight for independence and freedom of movement). I took the car keys on one of my visits and returned home having the peace of mind that she was safer because she could no longer drive her car. Well, I received a call I will never forget. She asked me, in a menacing tone, "Where are my keys?" I said, "Which keys are your talking about?" She said, "I'm not playing with you, bring me my G-D keys. I mean it!" Then she hung up the phone.

When You Got to Go. My mother was watching TV and got up to go upstairs. She stood at the bottom stair for about ten-seconds and did not go up. She walked over to a small trash can and placed it in the middle of the living room floor. She promptly stood in front of the can, pulled her underwear down and perfectly made a deposit in the can.

She then disposed of the contents and went back to the TV show. Great leg strength, balance and aim. The physical therapist would have been proud.

Hide and Go Seek and Seek and Seek. I checked areas around the house on a regular basis. This afforded me detection of behavior patterns, though I did not understand what I discovered. Prepare to be amazed at what you may discover, such as:

- Bedroom closets – hair rollers, knives, screwdrivers, single shoes, purses.

- Linen closet – one cooking pot, cornbread mix, more single shoes (with no laces).

- Dresser drawers – partial sandwiches, mail, glassware, silverware.

- Clothes hampers – soap, toothpaste, dustpan, canned food, trash.

- Between mattress and box spring – mail, checks, money, jewelry, food, tools, keys.

- Refrigerator – hair grease, toothbrush, TV remote, dish towel.

No Regard for Safety. Dementia seems to allow some urges to dominate thinking and behavior without regard for the associated dangers. My mother was a clean and orderly person. She would sweep her walkway and the sidewalk in front of her home. On occasion she would see debris in the street in front of her home and go out there and sweep. Drivers would stop with some being patient and others blowing horns. She would slightly move and adamantly wave them on as if she was the traffic officer, then return to sweeping.

Her Prerogative. I heard about this one, but it caught me really good. I was on my way for one of my mother's doctor visits. I had called her three times: one-hour, one-half hour and fifteen minutes prior to my arrival. She said she was ready, and I needed to get there. I came in the door to collect my mother and surprise!

She was dressed to impress with a nice blue top, slacks, shoes and hair somewhat combed. She also had on her nice white bra - over her top. In my mind I was saying, "Oh, heck no, we're not going out like that!" My higher mind just put a smile on my face and said, "That is a nice bra, how about you put it on the inside?" She said, "What's wrong with it the way it is?" I replied, "That's not the way you usually wear it and we have time for you to change."

She huffs, takes it off right there, and heads to the car. Oh, the looks I got walking up to, and into, the doctor's office. The doctor however said, "So, we are having one of *those* days." Yep, ladies' prerogative.

I Said I Was Cold. I am not sure if it is my mother, or the dementia, but she seemed cold during the summer months, August in particular. Seems her friends would visit often during the summer months. I appreciated that but felt sorry for them. I would come in the open door to find friends sweating with that, "Thank goodness you are here" look.

My mother complained she was cold and usually set the thermostat to 85 degrees. Her friends would make light mention of it but accepted that it was her home and she should be comfortable. I immediately turned the settings to 78 degrees seeking a happy medium. She jumped up as soon as she felt the cooler air and reset it to 85 degrees. The friends always said, "Thanks for trying."

Insight #5: *You will quickly find yourself experiencing headaches if you try to insist your dementia-stricken loved one should conform to your sense of normalcy.*

Insight #6: *You will need to develop diverse skills to compete against dementia.*

Reginald A. Lawson

CAREGIVER ROLES AND KEY FOCUSES

Adjust to what you are seeing and hearing.

"For the aged man is once again a child."

–Sophocles [c. 450BC] in Peleus

The dementia journey will introduce new experiences for you. Your functions, observations, and activities will need to change as your loved one progresses through their dementia stages. Here is my version of five roles and perspectives I suggest you consider adopting:

Caregiver Role 1: <u>Observer</u> for Dementia Stage: 2-3

- Caregiver Activity: Pay attention to slight forgetfulness, how they respond to forgetting, their language skills. Don't be critical or fearful of the forgetfulness.

- Real Life Phase Comparison: Think of someone in their 30s-50s, confident, very aware how things work, resourceful, and independent.

Caregiver Role 2: <u>Coach</u> for Dementia Stage: 3-4

- Caregiver Activity: Start giving guidance and direction; assess how well they perform and retain instructions; pay attention to their psychomotor skills, how they walk, hold a fork, write with a pen, hold papers closer to read, keep asking you to repeat yourself or to speak louder, increase in frustration.

- Real Life Phase Comparison: Think of someone in their teens-20s, trying to affirm their independence, pushing what they think works, questioning/struggling with why it does not work as they think it should.

Caregiver Role 3: <u>Director</u> for Dementia Stage: 4-5

- Caregiver Activity: This is where you need to have all authorities in place to handle financial, medical, and social decisions. You will need to protect them from themselves and their naiveté about the outside world. Delusions may start.

- Real Life Phase Comparison: Think of a pre-teen, rebelling and fighting to do what he wants to do while oblivious to the threats and consequences involved.

Caregiver Role 4: <u>Parent</u> for Dementia Stage: 5-6

- Caregiver Activity: You need to read body language better as verbal skills are diminishing; observe nervous energy and compulsive behavior. You would be wise to not try to control their behavior, just keep them safe; accept that things are getting worst and beyond your understanding.

- Real Life Phase Comparison: Think of someone 2-5 years old, having emotional bursts of laughter, crying, selfishness, idleness, increased sleeping, limited appetite; obstinate about doing the simplest things you ask of them.

Caregiver Role 5: <u>Sustainer</u> for Dementia Stage: 6-7

- Caregiver Activity: You will need to provide constant monitoring; they may barely get out of bed or eat more than 2-spoons of liquid, psychomotor skills are pretty much gone. Consult with Hospice Services.

- Real Life Phase Comparison: Think of the newborn infant struggling to manage the weight of their head, or eyes barely open; no words just grunts, if that; no control of bowels or swallowing.

A common mantra I received was, "Dementia will cause your mother to be mean." Great! She was already very good at that trait and they are telling me she will get worse.

Insight #7: *Take a moment and ponder the feeling of not being able to remember or recognize common things in your life. Try to remember that feeling. Your loved one has the right to be angry, which is how some people tend to handle being afraid.*

Reginald A. Lawson

DEMENTIA'S REROUTING GPS

Learn to pull over, park and listen.

Dementia will often cause your loved one to wander mentally. One of the constants about my mother was her frequent mental travels into her past. She seems to be able to recall, with clarity and deep emotion, events from teenage years, but not what transpired in the last 30 minutes. Our brain's structure and functions are fascinating, but I digress.

I found it helpful and learned so much about her childhood from listening to her concerns about family members. She was always saying she needed to go get her sister from getting into trouble at the dance hall or being out late. Seems her brother was her antagonist and she had to always put him into his place. She did not just remember these events—she was emotionally and physically reacting to those moments as if they were live.

These were stress-free moments. Be careful to not challenge them as to why they are talking about the past. Do your best to not insist they should, or have to, remember a certain person, place or thing: the harder you force this issue, the more anxious your loved one will become. Just let it be about them, wherever they are in that moment. Some of this journey may include delusions.

Just dance in the goodness of the moment as long as they seem safe. I would tell my mother that things would be just fine, and we would fix whatever was troubling her when she seemed worried. If their recollections are a little off or incorrect, so what?

Keep it about them and not about your understanding of the correct facts about a circumstance. So many things become temporary in their short-term memory. They will not be able to recall what they or you said once they enter into stage four.

Insight #8: *Let them have those rare and much needed peaceful moments.*

DISCOVERING THE GOODNESS WITHIN

Learn how to embrace the journey's rare sunshine.

You will be well served by arming yourself with a positive outlook on this journey. There will be enough challenges to your sanity. Many things do not repeat the same way. Do not spend time anticipating the negatives.

Please know that you matter, whether your loved one or anyone else tells you or not. Here are a few of the times I could find the *goodness* in the moment:

<u>Where's Harry?</u> My stepfather had passed, and my mother was a part of the full preparations for his farewell, at his home-going services and his internment. Her dementia had not presented itself that we could discern. However, in conversations with her, it became clear that her memory was getting worse. She asked from time to time "Where is Harry?"

In the beginning I said, "Harry passed away, don't you remember?" and she would angrily say, "No! When did it happen?" "Why didn't anybody tell me?" She would go sit alone sometimes with a tear and sometimes without. It would take her about ten months to stop asking "Where is Harry?" and instead ask "Is Harry dead?" I felt unjustified pains of guilt, as if I was causing her pain by taking him from her, each time I said, "yes he is."

The Goodness in this, before she could consistently remember, was that each evening she would smilingly say, "He better get home soon because I'm getting ready for bed." This was a sign of positive

expectations of an embrace to come, if but only in her mind.

<u>Donna King.</u> I recall coming in one day to visit my mother, a woman who took pride in her appearance, especially her silver hair. On this occasion she greeted me with straight, possibly finger-styled hair all over her head. I couldn't help but think, "Oh, she looks like Don King, the fight promotor."

Most importantly, she seemed to be her usual self and not bothered by the appearance. When family and friends inquired with, "How is your mother doing?" I would say, "She's in her Donna King moment".

The Goodness in this is, I was able to greet her with a smile thinking how her hair looked just like Don King's hair. Equally I realized that dementia freed her from frustration and embarrassment over her appearance because of her hair.

<u>Bus Stop People.</u> My mother liked to be outdoors. Getting her to go riding was easy on all but Bad Days. So off we would go to a park, appointments, or shopping. On occasion we would stop at a traffic light where there was a bus stop. 32Most of the time there were people waiting for the bus. My dear sweet mother would look over and get a sly grin on her face. Then she would say, "Look at those lazy 'so-in-soes', they need to be at work." I was shocked and appalled. My response was, "Mom those people aren't bothering you, leave them alone. They are waiting for the bus to get to work." She would usually start laughing and say something along the line of, "Then you should give them a ride."

The Goodness in this is, she was comfortable enough to express her emotions. My response let her know I also cared about others and would defend them. She would say, "You're a good person and I'm proud of

you." I would always respond, "Because you raised me that way."

Insight #9: *Take it one moment at a time. Find the goodness in each opportunity to experience the power of love. This is medicine for you—the Caregiver.*

Reginald A. Lawson

BECOMING SMARTER

Reginald A. Lawson

MIRAGES ON DEMENTIA'S HORIZON

Looking ahead at what is coming and how to prepare.

Dementia is personal, meaning two people with the same type will progress on their respective journeys at different paces. I am a problem solver and not afraid to face unknown circumstances or to learn new things. I learned and experienced, while serving as a State Trooper, that I belonged to a professional category, of risk takers, that does not handle deception very well.

This category includes trauma room personnel, people working with high power electricity, surgeons, fire fighters, to name a few. Caregiving can put a person into this category. We are ready to respond and need to trust that what we are facing to be true and stable as presented. Dementia can strike a blow when it takes over the sufferer's mind causing chaotic mirages thereby frustrating the caregiver's need for stability.

Dementia isn't a disease; it's a symptom. The term refers to a loss of brain function, as evidenced by memory loss, impaired judgment, behavior changes, learning difficulties, and communication problems.[2]

This dementia caregiving thing, I at first thought to myself, is a small logistical problem and it is just a matter of researching to find the solution. I was familiar with my mother's customary way of doing things. I knew her likes and dislikes, moods and values.

Here was my first mirage about the symptoms. My mother and I took a trip to see her brother. She traveled from her home in

Wilmington, DE, to BWI Airport, where I met her and that wonderful smile as she exited the Amtrak train. We soon boarded our flight to Detroit's Wayne County Airport. We arrived around 1 p.m. and enjoyed catching up with my uncle during the 30-minute drive to his home in Oak Park, Michigan, just outside Detroit.

We toured Detroit, had dinner and retired in my uncle's home around 10:30 p.m. with my mother's room next to mine. I awoke at 3 a.m. to find my mother looking puzzled while standing in my doorway. I asked her, "What was wrong" and she said, "Who moved my furniture?" I said, "This is uncle's house in Michigan." She said, "Don't tell me that, who moved my furniture!"

She began calling out loudly for her husband. I tried to calm her by explaining we were in her brother's home and flew there the day before. Her brother, hearing the commotion, joined us and asked her, "If she was alright?" My mother answered with, "I must be cracking up, I'm sorry for waking everyone." We laughingly dismissed it as a bad dream, and as something that happens with "getting older." The remainder of our three-day visit was uneventful. We flew back to BWI Airport, and she boarded the train for home and met her husband without any problems.

That event occurred 22 months before my mother was formally diagnosed. I had no clue that was a potential symptom of dementia. It gives me pause thinking about how she functioned to get off the train at the right stop both times. Angels were watching out for her.

Insight #10: *Initially, dementia offers subtle notices. It increases in frequency and intensity within a range of time.*

Insight #11: *I found it a helpful coping method to sometimes think I was traveling in a foreign country, needing to learn* *the language and customs of the people to be able to survive what I was going through on the journey.*

STAGES OF DEMENTIA

Mapping where you are on the journey.

You may hear dementia and Alzheimer's used interchangeably. Understand these are different things. Alzheimer's is the most common type of dementia. Here is a table to highlight some of the differences between dementia and Alzheimer's.[3]

	Dementia	Alzheimer's Disease
General Definition	A brain related disorder caused by diseases and other conditions.	A type of dementia. But the most common type.
Cause	Many, including Alzheimer's disease, stroke, thyroid issues, vitamin deficiencies, reactions to medicines, and brain tumors.	Unknown, but the "amyloid cascade hypothesis" is the most widely discussed and researched hypothesis today.
Duration	Permanent damage that comes in stages.	Average of 8 to 20 years.
Typical Age of Onset	65 years and older.	65 years but can occur as early as 30.
Symptoms	Issues with memory, focus and attention, visual perception, reasoning, judgment, and comprehension.	Difficulty remembering newly learned information. With advancement, disorientation, mood and behavior changes may occur.

Dementia vs Alzheimer's Disease

Do not just declare someone has dementia. A valid declaration requires testing by physicians. Common types of dementia include: [4]

1. Alzheimer's

2. Lewy Body Dementia

3. Vascular Dementia

4. Frontotemporal Dementia

5. Mixed Dementia

People with dementia may have problems with short-term memory, keeping track of a purse or wallet or keys, paying bills, planning and preparing meals, remembering appointments or traveling out of the neighborhood.

Stages of Dementia:

The Global Deterioration Scale (CGS) / Reisberg Scale [3], below, is widely accepted as a standard descriptor of the seven stages of dementia. Use the stages, diagnosis level, description of the signs and symptoms and the expected duration information as a reference point and not as absolutes.

Stage 1 – No Dementia Diagnosis – No Cognitive Decline

In this stage, the person functions normally, has no memory loss, and is mentally healthy. People with NO dementia would be considered in this stage. Duration is unknown.

Stage 2 – No Dementia Diagnosis – Very Mild Cognitive Decline

This stage is used to describe normal forgetfulness associated with aging. For example, forgetting names and where familiar objects were left. Symptoms of dementia are not evident to the individual's loved ones or their physician. Duration is unknown.

Stage 3 – No Dementia Diagnosis – Mild Cognitive Decline

This stage includes increased forgetfulness, slight difficulty concentrating, and decreased work performance. People may get lost more frequently or have difficulty finding the right words. At this stage, a person's loved ones will begin to notice a cognitive decline. Average duration of Stage 3 is between 2 years and 7 years.

Stage 4 – Early-Stage Diagnosis – Moderate Cognitive Decline

This stage includes difficulty concentrating, decreased memory of recent events, and difficulties managing finances or traveling alone to new locations. People have trouble completing complex tasks efficiently or accurately and may be in denial about their symptoms.

They may also start withdrawing from family or friends because socialization becomes difficult. At this stage, a physician can detect clear cognitive problems during a patient interview and exam. Average duration of Stage 4 is 2 years.

Stage 5 – Mid-Stage Diagnosis – Moderately Severe Cognitive Decline

People in this stage have major memory deficiencies and need some assistance to complete their daily living activities (dressing, bathing, preparing meals, etc.). Memory loss is more prominent and may include major relevant aspects of current lives. For example, people may not remember their address or phone number and may not know the time or day or where they are. Average duration of Stage 5 is 1.5 years.

Stage 6 – Mid-Stage Diagnosis – Severe Cognitive Decline (Middle Dementia)

People in Stage 6 require extensive assistance to carry out their Activities of Daily Living (ADLs). They start to forget names of close family members and have little memory of recent events. Many people can remember only some details of earlier life. Individuals also have difficulty counting down from 10 and finishing tasks.

Incontinence (loss of bladder or bowel control) is a problem in this stage. Ability to speak declines. Personality / emotional changes, such as delusions (believing something to be true that is not), compulsions (repeating a simple behavior, such as cleaning), or anxiety and agitation may occur. Average duration of Stage 6 is 2.5 years.

Stage 7 – Late-Stage Diagnosis – Very Severe Cognitive Decline (Late Dementia)

People in this stage have essentially no ability to speak or communicate. They require assistance with most activities (e.g., using the toilet, eating). They often lose psychomotor skills. For example, the ability to walk. Average duration of Stage 7 is 1.5 to 2.5 years.

My experiences deviated somewhat from the above time periods. I would guess we travelled in Stage 1 though Stage 3 for a duration of approximately 2 years. However, our duration from Stage 4 to Stage 7 was approximately 15 months. You should stay alert for signs of changes and take action. Procrastination can cause unnecessary challenges for everyone.

DEMENTIA PUNISHES PROCRASTINATION

If you can't, then find someone who can, but get this done!

There are wishes to be known and decisions to be made about support, decision-making authority, end-of-life management, and property. You should (will need to) address the realities of a diminishing quality of life for your loved one. Here are the key activities I am referring to when I say "address the realities":

1. A Medical Directive – to capture their wishes as to quality of living should their heart stop, or they suffer a stroke, i.e. do they wish to be dependent on a machine to keep them alive?

2. A Power-of-Attorney (POA) – to designate someone to handle their financial and medical decisions in the event they cannot make reasonable/rational decisions.

3. A Trust – to represent how their estate should be managed and by whom.

4. A Will – to decide key points in how they prefer to distribute their assets and possessions.

The most likely reality will be that your loved one will not want to address these things. The subject matter can serve as a reminder of something they, and possibly you, cannot handle well: the ending of their life.

Key Fact – Either you get this done before your loved one is declared to be of "unsound mind," or the State will decide all these things for you—period!

My timeline shows how close we came to not be able to represent and execute key decisions to keep my mother at home, pay her bills, obtain social services for her, or plan for her estate:

- May 9, 2011 – Executed Medical Directive.

- Aug 2, 2012 – Husband passes away.

- Aug 6, 2012 – Doctor Visit, doctor orders dementia test.

- Aug 7, 2012 – Executed POA, Trust & Will, my mother struggled to remember the day's date when signing the forms.

- Aug 10, 2012 – She cannot remember going to the attorney's office, his name or the passing of her husband.

- Aug 30, 2012 – Applied for Survivor Social Security benefits. My mother couldn't represent herself or remember her husband's passing from four weeks earlier.

Note: The Social Security Administration (SSA) did not honor the POA.

I was told, during our request for SSA benefits interview, that my mother had to answer for herself, therefore I could leave during the process. I smiled and suggested that I remain but said, "I would quietly set on the side." This was going to be one of those fun moments for me.

Still I Rise – Maya Angelou

The agent *finally* allowed me to get involved only after he was convinced that he could not get coherent answers from my mother. He asked me the questions and I asked my mother in a way I knew she understood.

Then I interpreted the answers for the agent. I know it sounds crazy, but it worked. Pack your patience and in this particular case have a copy of the marriage certificate and the spouse's death certificate. I suggest making copies (electronic usually works) of the above documents, as you will need to provide them in certain situations.

The following people or agencies wanted the Medical Directive:

- The medical professionals (doctors want one in their file

The following people or agencies wanted the POA in their files before they would discuss pre-death matters:

- Medical professionals (doctor, dentist, ER, pharmacist)
- Insurance company (life, health, auto and home)
- Current and former (if retired) employer
- City, county and state governments
- Utilities, cable and phone companies
- Credit card services will want one for their files
- Funeral service providers
- Your family (and possibly their attorneys)
- Case workers, Medicare, Medicaid want to see the documents

- Banks will need to see it, then execute one of their own to put on file (get a copy of their POA)

The following people or agencies wanted the Trust before they would discuss post-death matters:

- Medical professionals

- Insurance company (life, health, auto & home)

- Current and former (if retired) employer

- City, county and state governments

- Utilities, cable & phone companies for their files

- Credit card services

- Banks

- Funeral service providers

- Your family (and possibly their attorneys)

- Case workers, Medicare, Medicaid want to see the documents

The following people or agencies wanted the Will for post-death matters:

- City, county and state governments

- Your family (and possibly their attorneys)

I created a PDF of each and loaded them on my phone. This allowed me to immediately send them when speaking on the phone with an agency that needed one on file before they could speak with me. It also was convenient to be able to use their printer (via wireless network) to print off the documents as needed in their office.

You would be smart to understand the difference between "revocable" and "irrevocable" as applied in the State where the trust document is executed.

In brief, "a revocable living trust is a type of trust that can be changed at any time. An irrevocable trust is simply a type of trust that can't be changed by the grantor after the agreement has been signed and the trust has been formed and funded. For the most part, it is forever."[5]

Insight #12: *Get this done by the start of stage three! Having the above documents made quality decisions possible.*

YOUR FIRST RESEARCH PROJECT

Your road map for the halfway mark of the journey.

One of the smartest things you can do is find out what and who represents your loved one's assets, liabilities, services, programs, commitments and memberships. Here is a sample list.

Bank Account(s)
Who:
Identifier:

Life Insurance(s)
Who:
Identifier:

Auto Insurance
Who:
Identifier:

Health Insurance
Who:
Identifier:

Investments
Who:
Identifier:

Employer Pensions
Who:
Identifier:

Loans
Who:
Identifier:

Credit Cards
Who:
Identifier:

Subscriptions
Who:
Identifier:

Dentist
Who:
Identifier:

Physician
Who:
Identifier:

Pharmacies
Who:
Identifier:

Hairstylist
Who:
Identifier:

Church Committees
Who:
Identifier:

Civic Memberships
Who:
Identifier:

Cleaners
Who:
Identifier:

Lawncare
Who:
Identifier:

Mortgage
Who:
Identifier:

Tax Preparer
Who:
Identifier:

Legal Counsel
Who:
Identifier:

Cable/Internet
Who:
Identifier:

Telephone/Cell
Who:
Identifier:

Pest Control
Who:
Identifier:

Insight #13: *My best resource was my mother's five years' worth of checkbook ledgers. Also look in bibles or safety deposit box for documents.*

PULLING OVER – NOT SURE I CAN DRIVE

My driving skills were not working on this pothole riddled road.

I heard of caregivers' support groups, but I wanted to try it myself first, then get help if I could not figure it out. (Yes, I tend to look at the picture and start, then read the instructions as needed.) I was confident that I have a few approaches that should work right-away and give us a smooth ride. Wow, I immediately started praying for my tires to hold up as I hit pothole after pothole on this dementia road.

I am an advocate of medical-alert-jewelry. The challenge I ran into was my mother would not wear her jewelry consistently. I would ask, each time I visited, for her to put the medical alert bracelet on. She would ask me to put it on her. I thought this to be, at first, cute, then lazy, then resistant. I later considered that she could not put it on by herself. She never admitted it to me. Then it disappeared one day. That's right: It was hidden or stored away for safe keeping.

I would not even go the "Help, I've fallen" jewelry route. My mother had a curiosity that I am sure would have prompted her to press that button over and over. I should have received a heap of gratitude from the services that never had to respond to all those potential false alarms she would have surely caused.

Another option that failed to work were GPS-sneakers. These shoes are embedded with a chip that communicates with a satellite to give location information. This becomes invaluable should your loved one wander off. I purchased a pair and got my mother to wear them. We walked up and down her street, around the corner, drove to the mall and walked around, and then drove to a local park. The signaling from the satellite service to the app on my phone worked perfectly. **All set!**

She stopped wearing the sneakers about three weeks later. She also hid one of the sneakers and removed the shoelaces. That was a three-hundred-dollar, non-refundable lesson.

Adult Daycare was another failed venture. These programs are setup to provide your loved one with a fun-focused social outing during the day. You just contact your local government or senior services program coordinator to get started. A van or small bus usually comes to the house to pick up and return your loved one.

I highly recommend you plan to take them on a pre-program visit for about an hour—you will thank me later. Most places offer a tour or trial day to get you and your loved one familiar with how it looks and feels. We visited three programs. **Note:** Make sure you ask them about their leaving early policy.

All programs told me they would not change their departure schedule and my mother would have to wait it out if she wanted to leave early. I asked what if she just walked out the door? All of the programs stated, "We lock our doors for security purposes." This is a great precaution. However, I could envision my mother fighting to insist they let her go home.

Here I am, on our third program site visit, being pleasant and encouraging about the people of similar age, the group activities and lunch. My dearest mother says, "I don't want to be around all these sick-looking people, if you like it so much, then you stay, I'm going home." *That's not dementia, that is my mother, truth teller!*

At this point I do not know which direction to go next. Something has to change, and I know dementia is not volunteering to help. Let's try getting out the vehicle, walk around and then sit back in the driver's seat and pray for an inspiration or a useful perspective.

SHIFT TO DISCOVERY MODE

It helps a lot to understand their realities.

These are things no one told me to expect. I am going to tell you—because I truly believe having a heads-up before it happens will help bring you back from disbelief. Here you are, finally, thinking you are getting a handle on this thing and what you have come to accept as "normal," and they change.

How do I keep my composure while providing help to a grown person who has moments of childish behavior (like a 3-year-old with moodiness, tantrums, and sometimes unbridled confidence), quality-of-life challenges and a strong need to maintain their dignity?

Often you cannot learn of a true status about your loved one's needs because they mask them from you. This is usually out of pride, embarrassment, fear, or frustration. This can be so exasperating. Please remember, in the early stages they are cognizant of, and fighting, their reality. They get frustrated with not remembering where they placed something. Then in later stages they get embarrassed because, for instance, they have not properly interpreted a signal for a bowel movement.

They are so determined to hold onto their independence. These things are scary to them, as it would be to most of us. I found it best to approach this in *discovery mode*. Observe your loved one without the interference of focusing on who they were (the pre-dementia version). This needs to be a stealthy observation.

I believe one of the effects of dementia is heightened suspicion of others and that means our loved one is always checking others out. If they believe you are tracking them or trying to control them, then it is "game on." They will work even harder to hide the progression of the illness.

Remember they are aware of the impacts of dementia for most of the journey. It frustrates them that they are forgetting thoughts, names, and general understandings about the way things work—from remote controls to toilets. It scares them that they are losing control. They have their pride, dignity and independence they are fighting to keep them intact. Telling others of their fears and losses can be embarrassing and devastating to what little sense of self remains, so they try to keep it within.

I was fortunate to have a rare and insightful conversation with my mother about her feeling/reliving fears of her past. This conversation came on the heels of seeing her going back and forth with a worried and determined look scanning the room. If you have watched a dog scurrying around with a treat that they want to save (hide) for later, you know what I mean.

I asked, "Is something wrong, what can I help you do?" She responded, "That her first husband keeps stealing her money and she needed to hide it." For my mother, it did not matter, in that moment, that her first husband had passed away some eight years earlier. Key in on the three trigger words in my question: "wrong," "help," and "you." These words seem to improve her cooperation.

Insight #14: *Sometimes they will be defiant and declare nothing is wrong, and other times they will tell you. Don't get angry, because this is a real struggle for them. Sometimes it helps to relax your fear when the road gets bumpy because the vibration is temporary. Pause and retry.*

60

ADJUSTING YOUR FOCAL POINT

It works much better when you make it about them and not about you.

The following successes are the results of trial and error in an effort to cope with diverse and ongoing scenarios. Remember, your loved one is the person directly suffering the scary realities of dementia and will get defensive quickly on those Bad Days.

These are things you may face on a regular basis. I found that your mindset makes the difference in life. How you look at things (lens) and interpret things (perspective) will influence (suggest) the decisions you make and methods you use. The suggested mindset is to keep it light and supportive. The strategy is to try and put most of the situation on you, thereby reducing their guilt, embarrassment, and or anger about something they cannot control.

These are what finally worked for me for most of the journey (stages), especially on some of those Bad Days. I learned to have the following responses to things my mother said or did:

1. "I don't need a doctor / Why do I have to go to a doctor?"

    *   Old Response: "Because you have dementia and need to get checked."

    *   New Response: "I need to go for a quick visit and want you to come with me."

2. "We can't leave until I find my keys (that she keeps hiding)."

   - Old Response: "You need to stop hiding things, now we are going to be late."

   - New Response: "It's ok, I have my keys, so we can get back in the house."

3. "This is not my house."

   - Old Response: "Yes, it is, you have lived here 20 years."

   - New Response: I created and placed 5x7 cards in my mother's living room and bedrooms saying, "This is Gloria's house."

4. Mirrors covered up (my mother did not recognize herself and got scared):

   - Old Response: "Why do you have the mirrors covered/ turned away!?"

   - New Response: I placed happy pictures of my mom on the mirrors and walls.

5. "Did I ask you that already?"

   - Old Response: "Yes, six times, can't you remember?"

   - New Response: "Yep, you sure did, want to hear the answer again?" or just change the answer (to preserve your sanity).

6. "Why can't I remember things?"

   - Old Response: "Because you have dementia and it's doing it to you."

   - New Response: "You do remember (suggestive), it just takes a little longer to show up."

7. "Who's gonna stay with me?"

   - Old Response: "I can't stay - you'll be fine alone."

   - New Response: "Well, I need to go to work and will be back afterwards."

8. "Why can't I drive!?"

   - Old Response: "Because, you'll get into an accident!"

   - New Response: "The car is not safe to drive. I'm trying to get it fixed, but it will take a while."

9. "You don't tell me what to do. Who do you think you are!?"

   - Old Response: "Well you act like a child," or "You don't know what you're doing", or "I'm the one taking care of you."

   - New Response: "I'm sorry, I was afraid you would get hurt" or "I was trying to be helpful."

10. "I don't want to," or "Why do I have to, take that medicine, it makes me sick?"

   - Old Response: "Because you will get worse if you don't."

   - New Response: "I'm sorry about that. It is supposed to help you get healthier. I have to talk to the doctor to see if we can change them. OK?"

11. "Why do I need to sign that [Directive, Power-of-Attorney, Will]?"

   - Old Response: "Because if you don't, then the state will take everything."

   - New Response: "We need to legally represent your wishes to help avoid fighting the government/family."

B.A.G. DEMENTIA DAYS

Getting smarter at reading the signs.

You will learn that a straight logical approach will often fail you. You must learn how to navigate through dementia's curves and how to see and avoid its potholes. Finally, you must become a wise and resourceful traveler to handle the diverse types of dementia days. Frustration will give way, as you get better at doing this, to rewarding results for everyone.

I heard it said that there are three kinds of dementia days: bad, average, and good. A strategy for the caregiver may be to view those days as follows:

- Bring out your goodness on their Bad Days (B)

- Appreciate them on their Average Days (A)

- Celebrate with them on their Good Days (G)

The following are actual reactions depending on whether it was a Bad, Average, or Good Dementia Day:

Morning Waking (6 a.m.-7 a.m.):

- (B) Irritated by the cheerful greeting of the caregiver.

- (A) Feeling stiffness in her back slowing her initial movement.

- (G) Smiling as she listens to the birds.

Bathroom Visit (7 a.m.-7:30 a.m.):

- (B) Frustrated she can't remember how to flush the toilet.

- (A) Using a warm washcloth to clean up in the sink.

- (G) Face is clean, and hair is combed.

Breakfast (8 a.m.-8:30 a.m.):

- (B) Not willing to eat, irritated with whatever is in front of her.

- (A) Eating slowly or picking at food sometimes.

- (G) Polish off everything on the plate, moves it to the sink, wants to wash it.

In the House:

- (B) Pacing back-and-forth in sundowning mode (increased confusion and anxiety that arise late in the day).

- (A) Sitting watching TV.

- (G) Humming and taping or dancing.

Out of the House:

- (B) Fussing with small kids, animals.

- (A) Smiling at small kids, little eye contact with adults.

- (G) Enjoying sunshine, fresh air and music in the car.

Evening (6 p.m.-9 p.m.):

- (B) Rummaging through closets and drawers.

- (A) Standing staring out the window or front door.

- (G) Laughing at a TV show.

Retiring (9 p.m.-11 p.m.):

- (B) Pacing from bedroom to bedroom, annoyed by the sounds outside.

- (A) Standing staring out the window, then lying down.

- (G) Turning out the light, getting under the covers, and going straight to sleep.

Through the Night (11 p.m.-6 a.m.):

- (B) Timidly and repeatedly going from the bedroom to the hallway.

- (B) Looking down the stairs.

- (B) Going in and out of another bedroom repeatedly.

- (A) Getting out the bed to stare out the window then back in repeatedly.

- (A) Getting into a new bed.

- (G) Getting up to go to the bathroom.

- (G) Getting back into the same bed.

- (G) Resting.

_Insight #15__: A Bad night usually led to a Bad morning and continued until she got exhausted and took a nap. I usually talked to her, by phone, on those days during stage three, to reassure her that things would be better. However, she would self-correct most times in stage four, possibly because she could not remember what was bothering her the night before._

TIPS ABOUT YOUR IN-HOME SERVICE TEAM

Making at home care more manageable.

One of the challenges you will encounter is your loved one's unwillingness to go out, because they may develop fears of people and things. You also may not want to go out with your loved one due to their aggressive public behavior toward you or others. As much as we want to be patient with those we love and try to put their needs ahead of our own, it can be humiliating to be dressed down without reason in front of others.

You must, no matter the embarrassing circumstance, have key medical services for proper caregiving. A viable solution is to bring the needed services to the home. Some traditional out-of-the home services can be performed at home. This would help avert social awkwardness, and it will be great for giving yourself a needed break.

Screen all prospective providers for any experience they have had with people suffering cognitive decline. They will spend a lot of time alone with your loved one. Insist on meeting each person that will come in contact with your loved one and the home.

Focus on their temperament, as a positive one will serve everyone well. This includes the provider's staff, helpers or surrogate team. My mother liked to inject herself into whatever went on in her home. They were to call me immediately if her meddling became too hard for them to cope with and got in the way of them carrying out their duties. Most providers understood and co-existed well.

Everyone entering my mother's home was notified, via signs in the windows next to the doors, about our usage of cameras for her safety. Only one contractor declined to work in her home due to the cameras.

I told the providers to mind their tools, language and patience. One general contractor had to learn the hard way. My mother became friendly with him sharing smiles and small talk. He said she reminded him of his mom. One day he needed to go to his truck for a quick moment to get a tool. He returned to find his light pen and a couple wrenches missing. He learned!

Here are some of the services I used:

Primary Physician Team: If you can, find a team that will actually visit your loved one at home. The primary physician came every third visit and her assistants came all other times. This was so helpful, because:

- It eliminated the need for my mother to get dressed to go out.

- She was not exposed to the weather.

- We didn't have to deal with traffic or the unpredictability of events outside the home.

- I didn't have to negotiate with her about going to the doctor.

Podiatrist: Think of this as a pampering moment. Our podiatrist had a soft personality and helped reveal and reduce pains from foot issues my mother could not remember and therefore, did not speak about.

X-ray Technician: This was priceless. There was no need to go sit in a waiting room or contend with issues (lashing out at, or fearful of, other people). They just lay down on their bed and relax while the technician takes X-rays.

<u>Music Therapist</u>: This is an absolute must—if you can get one. There are several studies about the influences these therapists can have on improving the quality of living in the moment. Just tell the therapist, in advance if possible, the type of music your loved one likes or grew up listening to.

<u>Physical/Occupational Trainer</u>: They help assess and improve movement. This group sees hip movement, walking gait and other possible weak postural issues. You can get some targeted at-home exercises to help keep your loved one safer.

<u>Food Delivery:</u> There are some great ways to supplement food for your loved one. Research grocery delivery, fast-food delivery, and social programs delivery. I used Meals-On-Wheels. This worked for most of the stages of my mother's dementia.

However, they stopped bringing the food in the home and she started not opening the door. Their policy stated, "If two deliveries are not accepted (by someone to receive the food) then the service is cancelled."

<u>Home Cleaning:</u> This is another valuable service. You need to set this up carefully. The notion of having strangers going through the house can be unsettling.

Having the service providers address her with respect (as Ms. G) worked like a charm. On the third visit she just opened the door and sat back down throughout the service.

In-home cleaning agencies experience high personnel turnover. You will most likely have a different team show up on the next appointment. Their focus is to provide you a service and not a particular person or team each time.

You can insist or ask but may find choosing an independent team (let's say husband and wife team, or one-person team) is the better solution to achieve continuity.

<u>Lawn Care and Snow Removal Service:</u> This was critical for us. My mother liked to do her own gardening. She could not keep up with the needed schedule for lawn care.

Additionally, she would forget to turn the water off after watering the lawn and plants (a $300 water bill).

I decided to replace the grass with mulch and some colorful bushes, including some double knockout roses. We had no grass cutting, fertilizing or watering to be concerned about. She loved it.

In the beginning my mother would not venture onto the snow-covered walkway; however, this changed as she got worse. Your concern should always be their safety.

Insight #16: *Plan to start in-home services in stage four.*

Insight #17: *The Music Therapist may create a playlist for you, or you can create your own. I used the playlist every-time we went driving. Oh, happy day!*

Insight #18: *Plan to be there the first two to three visits to ensure everyone is comfortable about the service. Your loved one may rebel and follow or attack the provider.*

Insight #19: *Select a service that understands your situation (a loved one with dementia) and ask them to try to service your needs early in the day.*

BEWARE OF SMILING FACES – A RARE INSIGHT

Trust your loved one's instincts about their potential caregivers.

The paid caregivers always presented a smiling, confident and flexible demeanor when I was there. The following was a wakeup call I received from reviewing footage captured by my kitchen safety camera. I do not believe I would have adequately understood the depth of the matter had I been present.

One day my mother got fed up with the level of service from her paid caregiver. I watched my mother look over at the caregiver who was watching some video on her phone. My mother had that look! She got up and went to the back door and paused.

Once she heard the caregiver start walking towards the back, about two minutes later, my mother went out the back door. The caregiver told her she needed to come back in, and my mother complied. My mother challenged her as to why she needed to come in since she is a grown woman, and this was her house. The caregiver said, "Because I want you to stay in." My mother smirked and went to sit back down.

Ten minutes later the same thing happened, but this time my mother went out the front door and down the street. I called my mother once they returned to the house, and the caregiver answered saying, "It is good you called because your mother is having a bad day." I asked my mother "If she was feeling OK and how things were going?"

She said, "Things are going good, but I am not going to have you paying good money for her to sit up here on the phone all day. So, I am making her work and hope she gets sick of it and quits." I said, "I love you and I will start looking for a better person today."

Insight #20: *Despite her dementia, my mother had sense enough to know whether a caregiver was delivering the services she was being paid to provide or just biding her time and collecting a paycheck for watching videos on her phone.*

CHOOSING THE RIGHT PAID CAREGIVER

Getting ready for one of your most important decisions.

The need for experienced paid caregiving (PC) will arrive. There are agencies and independents. Some agency members will do independent work, just ask. **Check references from actual clients, not family and friends**!

They all provided hourly rates, with a minimum number of hours. You may initially need them just a few hours and days, but this will increase. Budget for change in the scope of work. Some PCs will negotiate cost if they can get a long-term commitment from you. I know "long-term" is a relative term given what you will be managing. It helps them to know you are a steady and reliable client. Plan to do trial sessions, say three.

Here are the questions and answers I found as good indicators of a possible good fit for our needs:

* Have you been trained in dementia care? (A yes is the answer you want to hear.)

* How many years have you been providing dementia care? (Two years should be the minimum.)

* Where have you worked with dementia patients? (Institutional work involves working with multiple patients and having other dementia patients coming into spaces taking things from one another. There are also additional caregivers to help in the moment. Private home experience involves lesser immediate

additional caregiver support if a patient becomes a challenge.)

- How many dementia patients have you work with? (The higher the number the better.)

- How many clients do you have right now? (The more clients they have, the less ability they have to provide you more time when your care needs increase.)

- How have you handled a combative patient? (Do they talk to them, or try to physically constraint them, or ignore them?)

- How do you encourage a patient to eat when they don't want to eat? (Do they use guilt or fear, or do they treat them like a child, or just leave the food?)

- Do you have a backup caregiver for emergencies? (A yes is the answer you want to hear.)

- Do you cook, and if so, which oils and seasoning do you use? (Consider how their cooking style will complement or conflict with what is customary or needed for your loved one.)

- How do you travel—public transportation, personal vehicle, or do they depend on rides from others? (How will they get to the home in inclement weather?)

Insist on interviewing the backup caregiver once you make a hiring decision. You decide if the backup is acceptable or not. Listen to your loved one's comments about the PCs. People are usually attentive and polite in the beginning, but their true colors begin to show the more time they spend caregiving.

Make sure you read the caregiver's contract, whether agency or independent, to confirm the following key points at a minimum:

- Whose insurance provides for the PC should an injury occur?

- Can the PC eat portions of the food you brought, and they prepared for your loved one?

- Do you expect the PC to do the shopping, laundry or light cleaning?

- Do you want the PC to take your loved one out (walks, shopping, doctor's visits)?

- Do you want daily, weekly and/or significant issues updates?

- Can the PC decide who comes and goes in the house?

- Can the PC have guest, for them, at your loved one's home?

- How is a replacement or termination handled?

My mother and our first caregiver had a conversation in the kitchen one morning. My mother had an edgy tone and told the caregiver, "You don't have to be here, and you can go!" The caregiver said, "I'm being paid to be here and put up with your stuff." If there is low-to-no comfort level with your caregiver, then replace them! Getting the right one is priceless. Your loved one will feel safer and you will feel relieved.

Insight #21: *Interview for your loved one's particular condition. Ask questions about Alzheimer's if that is your circumstance. Ask about dementia if that is the case. Ask about bi-polar if that is your case.*

Insight #22: *I am a strong advocate for using cameras to alert you to what your loved one is experiencing. I learned a disturbing truth while reviewing footage one day.*

Insight #23: *If you have a bad feeling about a caregiver, or if you started out feeling confident with your choice but notice that you're getting a different vibe than you initially did, don't hesitate to trust your gut.*

BECOMING SAFER

Reginald A. Lawson

NEEDING BETTER ANSWERS

Making decisions from facts, not opinions or guesses.

All my suggestions about why and how you might want to detect and respond to your loved one's ability to handle everyday situations are experience-based. These are the things it took me a long time to understand and improve. The sooner you can discern changes in behavior, the sooner you can provide better protection from the associated threats.

You will be asked several questions once you consult with professionals who are familiar with dementia. They will need to assess where your loved one is along the continuum.

Here is a sampling of the questions:

- Can they remember who you are?

- Are they sleeping well?

- Do they have regular bowel movements?

- What and when do they eat?

- Do they close their house doors or leave them open?

- Do they go outside?

- Are they dressing appropriately?

- Can they still cook or heat up food?

Your answers will influence selected approaches with regard to safety. The nature of dementia can make information gathering difficult because it causes them to forget an event occurred.

Your best and primary source, under normal circumstances, is the loved one suffering with dementia.

When they do remember, dementia will rob their memory of all the facts. The worst-case scenario is when they are explaining an event, with conviction, that turns out to have been a dementia-induced hallucination. That's when it becomes necessary to enlist other people in the information-gathering process.

Insight #24: *Gather as much accurate data as possible to heighten the creditability and value of the given information, which will improve the positive impact of your chosen approach.*

AWARENESS

Learning about the realities of your dementia journey.

There are several things to consider with anyone being home alone. Once I understood that dementia is unique for each sufferer, I knew I needed to understand how it was impacting my mother. I had requests, in addition to my own curiosity, from medical teams, social services and family and friends about my mother. I had to accept that I would not know everything. I started out by doing what I always did—have conversations in person and on the phone with my mother. The answers were easy in the early stages of dementia when her memory was strong and allowed her to be very accurate. My challenge was that I lived two-hours away and needed more data. It was clear I needed to enhance my approach to give me more confidence and comfort in keeping her at home safely. I decided to pull in surrogate eyes and ears. I asked visiting family to share what they saw on visits, and what they heard on phone calls. I asked other visitors to share their experiences with my mother's behaviors and their observations on her levels of conversation and memory.

This seemed like a great approach, and it worked, until:

- the visits reduced,

- the helper became overwhelmed by the experience, or

- they kept insisting I put her away.

I am very thankful for everyone's support. However, it was a mistake to think what we saw was sufficient once she entered into stage three and beyond. Her recall skills diminished.

Think of the iceberg, there is much more to it than what you see above the surface. The key was to collect and analyze valid data across time and space. My mother's dementia provided some degree of predictability once I studied her patterns. My personal and professional backgrounds taught me to use triage-type approaches:

- Data, Information, Intelligence

- Detect, Execute, Evaluate

- Prevent, Mitigate, Survive

I believe in testing outcomes to verify their dependability. Your loved one is counting on you to get it reasonably right. Confirm your assumptions and increase peace of mind for all concerned.

Insight #25: *I divided my safety focus into three areas 1) health; 2) in the home; and 3) outside the home.*

MEDICATION SAFETY

Sometimes the best medicine is no medicine.

The doctor's honesty and openness were refreshing and the most helpful. She told me the following in clear terms:

"What will most likely cause your mother's death will be the brain forgetting how to swallow due to complications of dementia"

—Dr. Debrah Zarek (mom's first physician)

I accepted the doctor's frank words and decided to commit to improving my mother's "quality of life" up until that transition time. The doctor did as most doctors do—prescribed medicines. My mother was already taking medicine to address anemia, arthritis, high blood pressure, and low vitamin D. Now she would get medicine to address anxiety, improve sleep, and to slow memory loss. The doctor and pharmacist felt the drug interactions would be very safe.

The doctor asked for us to monitor:

- my mother's sleeping (whether she was getting enough rest through the night), and

- her bowel movements (whether they were productive and frequent). More on this in the Scenarios, Strategies and Tactics Section.

It seemed her anxiety might fluctuate, and impact sleep and she might become constipated. We used a weekly pill box, to manage distribution, since different people helped out and we did not want to miss a dosage. Easy as pie, she got the dosage consistently and on-time.

However, my mother complained about stomach pains after taking her twice-a-day grouping. She also seemed drowsy at mid-day. The doctor encouraged us to give her system a few more weeks to settle. She kept complaining. We (the doctor and I) reduced her dosage and frequency to the point of no medicine. Surprisingly this resulted in her having more energy, improved alertness and reduced complaints of pain.

Insight #26: *Once she entered into stage three, I changed the location of the medicines so that she would not have direct access to them, only designated helpers knew of the new placement.*

IN AND AROUND THE HOME SAFETY

Revealing the dementia-induced dangers in plain sight.

Here are, given my experiences, minimal in the home situations to assess and make decisions on. Remember you will need to adjust your detection and preventive measures as the dementia gets worse. You would be prudent to fully implemented these measures by stage four. **Note:** Do not expect your loved one to be able to tell you they are struggling. They may not remember having an issue or may be embarrassed to admit it.

Sharp Items: Absolutely remove these in stage four. I'll make this one simple, would you trust a 5-year old with knives, screwdrivers, scissors, or box cutters? You must search for these items throughout the entire house. I declare that dementia gave my mother unreal abilities to hide things so well that I could not find in my first or second search. Persevere so that you can find and remove these things.

Lighting: Your loved one can all-of-a-suddenly express challenges with the brightness of a light. High ceiling lighting helps illuminate an area to improve the ability to see obstacles and locate items. This works well until they complain that the lighting is too bright. Somehow, their processing of the light changes and it becomes uncomfortable. Lower the light some, then check again in one day or two days to see if that was an improvement. Some bulbs give off a low ringing or slight humming sound. This becomes increasingly irritating as the dementia progresses. Change the bulbs when they complain about hearing a ringing, just in case it is coming from the bulbs.

<u>Vision:</u> Something happens to challenge their depth perception. This becomes a threat when they cannot distinguish the depth of the floor in front of them. A throw rug of a contrasting pattern or color may create the illusion that one section of the floor is higher or lower than the others. This will quickly erode their confidence in going through an area. You have to pay attention, because they may not say a word, but will take evasive measures, for instance avoiding that area or treading very gingerly.

<u>Footing:</u> I found, during stage four, my mother slightly dragged her left foot. She began stumbling on the throw rugs. Needless to say, that increases the risk of falling. This is an easy fix: Remove the throw rugs. Another thing to consider is footwear. My mother preferred to wear socks half the time. People with dementia can lose or misinterpret sensory from their feet. I replaced her regular socks with socks having a rubber pattern on the bottom, like those hospitals provide to patients that are at risk of failing or slipping. I also installed anti-slip strips on all staircases. This helps if they have wet footwear. These can be a pain to clean, but that inconvenience is far better than the pain my mother would have suffered from a fall.

<u>Chemicals:</u> Again, this is a stage four alert, when the ability to properly interpret things start diminishing. Their sense of taste and what it means changed in potentially dangerous ways. I include in this group soaps (hard and liquid), bath oils, cleaners (floor, polish), and sprays (windows, cooking oils, pesticides, perfumes/cologne). What alerted me to this danger was going into my mother's bathroom to wash my hands. Right there was a bar of soap with teeth marks on it. A look into the cabinet revealed two more soap bars with teeth marks.

<u>Door Locks:</u> I strongly suggest getting coded door locks. This removes the challenge of looking for, or worrying about, keys. You do not need a locksmith to install most of these locks. Get the ones that allow at least ten codes to be assigned. I selected one that provided thirty codes. I assigned a master code, sub-master code, frequent family member codes, medical team codes, and contractor codes.

I also created five one-time codes (they are deleted once used) for emergency personnel such as police, fire, and EMS/EMT. The code assigning gave selective access to certain people and it logged their usage. This helped me cross-reference who visited and when. I could even tell when one member used someone else's code. The added security allowed me to remotely suspend or delete a code should someone need to be kept out.

<u>Mail Delivery:</u> Change their mail delivery.

1. They will lose the ability to distinguish a bill from a solicitation for money.

2. They will discard important information, i.e. notices, tax bills, and warranties.

3. They may become afraid of, or want to go out with, the mail delivery person.

I submitted a change of address form with the US Postal Service (the "change period of redelivery" has a time limit). Then I changed the mailing address with the various senders. This also allowed for cancellation of unnecessary subscriptions. I did allow AARP magazines delivery because she enjoyed them. Simply **put the subscription in your name, but for your loved one's address**, so it does not get caught up in the change-of-address process.

<u>Telephone:</u> Change their phone number to your name. Also, setup and review their Caller ID because:

1. You can detect solicitation calls and block them.

2. You can setup do not disturb times per their sleep periods.

3. You get immediately notification if there is an outage.

I noticed, as I zoomed closer with the kitchen camera, that my mother had removed the entire phone junction box, not the jack, from the wall. She told me, "The darn thing kept ringing during her T.V. soap operas." Time to call the general contractor, again.

I considered cancelling her number, but that would mean family, friends and social services (check-on-the-welfare type programs) would not be able to talk to her. However, I highly recommend, once they get to stage four, or cannot carry on a decent conversation, that you do have their calls forwarded to you. Change your voicemail to include something like: "You have reached voicemail for [your name] and your loved one's name." The other option is to set a voicemail for two months, then cancel the line.

Insight #27: *The US Postal Service kept delivering junk mail. You have to be exact about the addresses to include in your change form. Look at the addresses of all your loved one's mail and include "Current Resident" in the listing for redelivery.*

Insight #28: *Be careful about forwarding the phone calls to you. The first issue is that you will be unable to call your loved one, because their phone will ring back to you. Secondly, the increased calls on your phone may become annoying.*

OUTSIDE THE HOME SAFETY

Understanding how to travel safer with dementia.

Travel: Let's use the child scenario regarding going outside the home considerations. You want to minimize frustration for both of you. Here are some things to ponder:

- How long will you be traveling in the vehicle? Dementia can cause child-like restlessness or irritation from sitting in one place for a long period of time. You should pay attention during the early drive periods to get a sense of what "long time" is for your loved one. This time period most likely will shorten as the dementia progresses.

- What time of day and which route will you travel? Most of us get bothered by stop-and-go driving, even in good weather. I scheduled, when I could, appointments and outings to occur after rush-hour (heavy traffic times). I tried to avoid known road construction areas. You may have to endure the not-so-cute and repeated child-like, "Are we there yet?" question, or "Where are we going?" In worst case, they will start yelling at the other drivers.

- What type of environment will you spend most of your time visiting? Trips to food stores are usually comforting with the colorful displays and spacious walking aisles. But be mindful of extremely cold or warm indoor temperatures. My mother did not like the refrigerated sections. They may wander off to avoid cold areas.

- Trips to malls can be challenging because of the long walks from parking lots and garages, longer paths to get through the mall, and the crowds, along with the noise and visual discomfort of being surrounded by so many people.

Restroom needs are interesting. You may get one of two comments when they need to go to the rest room. The first comment may be, "Where's the bathroom?" The second comment goes like this, "I'm ready to go home now!" OK, outing is over and home we go.

How do you watch them when you need to go to the restroom? Here were my solutions:

- Take someone else with you to watch your loved one.

- Make eating the last part of your outing, then go home.

<u>Separation</u>: Remember you are their trusted guardian. Separation from you may become a disturbing issue beginning with stage four. They attach comfort to the familiarity of your face.

"Persons living with dementia can't remember, and often they have no concept of time. For example, sometimes I go to throw out the trash and Dotty will "accuse" me of having been gone for hours."[6]

Here are circumstances of natural separation, and the associated stage, that created a challenge for my mother and my adjustments:

- I would leave to go home for the night (stage four) and told her I would be back as soon as I could.

- I forgot something, went back into the house leaving her in the car (stage four). I asked her to stay and watch the car and I locked the doors (only if car is off).

- I would get out to pump gas (stage four) and told her to remain inside because the gas stinks.

- I would not risk separation for events where we are out of the house and she would be out of my eyesight, such as picking up prescriptions, clothes from cleaners, or mail from the post office, or going into a bank.

Energy: Get a feel for their energy cycle during the day. Do they have their best energy upon waking, or in the middle of the day or in the evening? Adjust your efforts and expectations to match their energy. Walk at their pace. Sit as long as they need to sit.

Insight #29: *In stages one through three I would just wait outside the restroom knowing she could handle the process. However, starting with stage four, the wait period became longer, and my concerns grew.*

Reginald A. Lawson

CELEBRATION CONSIDERATIONS

Learn how to manage celebrations in a positive manner.

We had family get togethers for Easter, Mother's Day, My Mother's Birthday, Thanksgiving and Christmas. Everyone wanted to include my mother in their celebrations, when it was their turn to host, as she was the de facto grandmother for the family.

Whoever was hosting called inviting me, because it was understood, if you wanted my mother to attend (post dementia diagnosis) you needed me to talk to her. My mother would say to me, "I'll go if you go."

Our general expectations were, my mother would enjoy the sight of family, young and old, and she would stay for a couple of hours. We learned that these expectations would be realized lesser and lesser as the dementia progressed.

I wish I had the following understandings during my mother's final years. These would have helped avoid some embarrassing and stressful moments. Read more about creating a safe and calm space.[7]

Consider these approaches to create an appropriate environment during the holidays for the person with dementia:

- <u>Tone down decorations.</u> Avoid blinking lights or large decorative displays that can cause confusion. Avoid decorations that cause clutter or require you to rearrange a familiar room.

- <u>Avoid safety hazards.</u> Substitute electric candles for burning candles. If you light candles, don't leave them unattended. Avoid fragile decorations or decorations that could be mistaken for edible treats, such as artificial fruits. If you have a tree, secure it to a wall.

- <u>Play favorite music.</u> Familiar or favorite holiday music may be enjoyable. Adjust the volume to be relaxing and not distressing.

To help the person with dementia enjoy the holidays:

- <u>Prepare together.</u> Invite them to help mix batter, decorate cookies, open holiday cards or make simple decorations. Focus on the task rather than the outcome.

- <u>Host a small gathering</u>. Aim to keep celebrations quiet and relaxed.

- <u>Avoid disruptions.</u> Plan a gathering at the best time of day for the person with dementia. Keep daily routines in place as much as possible.

- <u>Provide a quiet place</u>. If you are having guests over, provide a quiet place for the person with dementia to have time alone or to visit with one person at a time.

- <u>Plan meaningful activities.</u> You might read a favorite holiday story, look at photo albums, watch a favorite holiday movie or sing songs.

- <u>Keep outings brief.</u> If you'll be attending a holiday gathering, plan to be brief or be prepared to leave early if necessary. Make sure there is a place to rest or take a break.

- <u>Monitor Spatial Energy Levels.</u> Pay attention to increased movement, noise and volume of people around your loved one. They may become agitated, feel threaten or frighten and need to leave.

Insight #30: *What worked for us was an area where my mother could sit, like on a two-person couch, away from the loudest part, usually the kitchen, and play a video game. She could receive one visitor at a time, and she did not feel uncomfortable in that space.*

HELPING OUR FIRST RESPONDERS

Empower others to help your loved one in crisis.

I give profound thanks to all those who provide comfort and support to people suffering with dementia and their family members. These are the volunteer and paid caregivers, in-home contractors, Hospice workers, physicians, nurses, technicians, first responders, emergency room teams, home cleaning workers, and therapist.

Our first responders and emergency room personnel are highly trained in their specialties, unfortunately some have little patience when faced with uncooperative people. You can help them by providing a simple understanding that your loved one has cognitive challenges.

I attended a few dementia informational sessions with a panel that included emergency services presenters. Their presentation centered on some of the challenges they encountered when they responded to calls involving dementia sufferers.

Here are nine actual statements from the respective groups. I am providing my additional suggestions, in parentheses (), to offer alternative solutions for the presented problem:

From Fire Department Representatives:

- *"Have working smoke and carbon monoxide detectors on each level of the home."*

  (Traditional smoke detectors give off a piercing sound that will scare your loved one especially at night and in the dark. I chose talking smoke/carbon monoxide detectors that would provide voice warnings of what was going on, where it was being detected, and provide light and alerted me via text immediately.)

- *"In the event of a fire, we need access to the home."*

  (I replaced the standard key locks with automated coded locks. I created a one-time code for emergency personnel. I would contact the respective department if there was an alert and provide their code. That eliminated the need to break doors or glass for access.)

- *"Those with two-sided door locks need to leave the key in the lock or put it where it can be reached."*

  (Dementia suffers tend to move/misplace/hide things, especially keys. Once you move into stage five, I suggest dual coded locks [identical locks that fits both sides of the door] and installation of an emergency egress setup linked to the smoke detector. This will allow automatic unlocking of the locks.)

From EMS/ Ambulance Department Representatives:

- *"Create an emergency file/folder with key names, illnesses and contact information."*

  (Supplement this by having the information on your phone and the phones of other key points of contact. This allows quick and accurate recall, especially when you are panicked by the call at 2 in the morning.)

- *"Place the emergency file/folder on the refrigerator."*

  (This step can/will be easily defeated once the loved one gets hold of the folder. I suggest you put it either on top of the refrigerator or in a higher cabinet next to it. Do not let your loved one see you placing it there, or it will disappear.)

- *"Include a list of all medications and allergies."*

  (This is an absolute to provide, however the list may not be where you left it. I placed a sign [3x5 laminated card] in the front window and one taped onto the refrigerator instructing emergency services to call me in case of emergency. I kept the list on my phone allowing me to immediately tell [in-person or text] EMS, hospitals, pharmacies and doctors the requested information.)

From Police Department Representatives:

- *"Call as soon as your loved one is missing."*

  (Install cameras focused on the likely path your loved one will travel to leave the front and back property. Choose a camera that provides immediate alerts and fencing [virtual boundary marking] to detect when they leave. Now you can provide police with the time they left, direction they took, and attire.)

- *"Provide your loved one with a medical-emergency jewelry."*

  (Nice idea, but my mother said it bothered her and she kept taking it off. I chose the bracelet style out of concern for her cutting herself if she snatched a necklace off. We also placed emergency cards in purses and shoes and pinned them inside favorite coats. This of course only works if they wear these items.)

- *"Be ready to provide names and locations of places they may visit if wandering."*

(Dementia takes the mind into the past. My mother got to stage four and could not remember her house location standing thirty yards away.

Even if she wanted to go to her favorite place, she would not know where it was or how to get there on foot, let alone by car.

When you take them for a walk, or a drive pay close attention to places and things they start talking about with emotion. One day my mom did wander, and we found her two blocks away tired and sitting on a park bench, but not the park we usually visit across the street from her home.

Be prepared for these incidents, because dementia will cause the unexpected and unpredictable to happen.)

You have to make a fundamental decision on how to detect and respond to your loved one's safety needs. Monitored systems are fine, however, they are setup for ingress related events.

I needed a reasonably reliable way to help me improve:

- detection of something possibly wrong with her or in her environment

- how I could intervene to stop or reduce threats

- data I provided family, medical professionals and law enforcement, and

- how I could enhance future responses.

The resulting approach needed to help:

- reduce fears (mine and others)

- improve awareness (mine and others)

- improve responsiveness (mine and others)

- improve safety (my mother's and others while helping her), and

- allow us to get some needed rest (everyone).

What eventually worked was for me (not the paid alarm services) to do the monitoring, using compatible key products and apps with programmed auto alerts to my phone.

Insight #31: *Get a red cross seatbelt sleeve and fill-out the information card with your loved one's name and that they have dementia. Place it on their seatbelt each time they travel.*

DETECT AND PROTECT

Learning how to identify, detect and reduce threats.

This section discusses my implementation of automation and technology in my caregiving. I could not always be there to see and hear how my mother functioned through her day. I could, however, be there in a virtual way.

The implementation and integration of cameras, speakers, sensors, switches, locks and valves helped me to profile my mother's movements and needs. That profiling gave me insights on sleeping and movement patterns. It gave more than just data. It gave real information that I used to get smarter about how to create a safer environment for her.

I share these approaches because they protected her from some of the vulnerability's dementia sufferers experience. It took me about three years to design, evolve and fine-tune what finally worked for us. The resulting system was not a perfect system for every scenario, but it positioned me to spare my mother actual and perceived harms.

I have started configuring and helping implement my system for others. The quicker you can supplement your caregiving, the sooner you can reduce some of your anxieties and doubts.

Read on to learn how I used technology to successfully address common and frequent scenarios associated with someone living at home with dementia.

Reginald A. Lawson

RECOMMENDED TECHNOLOGY

Improving your information gathering and decision making.

All of these suggestions will require an internet connection and the implementation of a central controlling device, usually referred to as a hub. Choose a hub that has flexibility to work well with peripheral devices such as sensors, cameras, alarms, outlets, switches, locks, light bulbs and motors. The hub provider will have a list of which devices are compatible.

Automation Hub

- Principal Purpose: Integrate various devices
- Primary Features: Compatible, battery backup
- Secondary Features: Works with your signal repeaters

Automated Video Doorbell

- Principal Purpose: Records who comes to the door
- Primary Features: Wireless, live viewing
- Secondary Features: Temporary storage

Camera for Indoors

- Principal Purpose: Detects location status and movement

- Primary Features: Night vision, 160 degree viewing angle

- Secondary Features: Speaker/microphone, pan/tilt/zoom

Camera Management Unit

- Principal Purpose: Controls viewing setup and camera movement

- Primary Features: Live viewing, footage storage

- Secondary Features: Upload stills and video, playback

Camera for Outdoors

- Principal Purpose: Detects location status and movement

- Primary Features: Night vision, 160 degree viewing angle

- Secondary Features: Speaker/microphone, zoom

Controllable Outlets

- Principal Purpose: Turns devices on and off

- Primary Features: Wireless

Door Locks

- Principal Purpose: Control entry and exit
- Primary Features: Programmable, battery powered, wireless signal (z-wave), activity logging
- Secondary Features: Auto-releasable switch

Light Bulbs

- Principal Purpose: Provide safe & supportive light
- Primary Features: Wireless
- Secondary Features: Dimmable

Light Switch

- Principal Purpose: Control lighting
- Primary Features: Wireless

Programmable Thermostat

- Principal Purpose: Control environment temps
- Primary Features: Wireless, programmable
- Secondary Features: Sends notifications

Sensor – Temp, Water

- Principal Purpose: Detect climate and leaks
- Primary Features: Wireless, battery-powered

Sensors – Motion, Status

- Principal Purpose: Detect movement, open/close status

- Primary Features: Wireless, battery-powered

Make sure you pay attention to the list designation. Some devices have been tested by the hub manufacture or independent labs and classified as "highly" compatible. Other devices that have not been classified as "highly", but "should be" compatible due to the type of technology that device uses (i.e. z-wave© ZigBee, wi-fi, etc.) usually work.

Review your internet parameters for speed. Most providers boast about download speed. Remember, most systems are setup for watching movies and playing game and not setup for monitoring a dementia sufferer. You will want upload speed for sending alerts, pictures, sound and video.

__Insight #32__: Warning: Systems such as Alexa should not be re-purposed as a dementia care safety system. These systems do not interface with automated locks and you do not want your demented loved one giving commands.

MY TECHNOLOGY SETUP

Technology is a tool, not a replacement for love.

The following describes how I configured my mother's automated detection system. Here were the logistics influencing my decisions:

- I could not be there 24/7.

- The quickest I could respond from home was two-hours.

- There were local, reliable service people to respond to non-mental issues.

These circumstances heighten the need for timely and accurate information to enhance decision-making. I needed to know:

- Where was my mother at any given time?

- What was she doing at any given time?

- Who was in her immediate space?

- Whether she was in imminent danger.

The smartest thing was to gather accurate data allowing me to alert, inform and direct the appropriate resources to help my mother. Sometimes issues where handled by a phone call to her, sometimes remotely activating a lock or light would suffice, and other times family, neighbors or emergency personnel would be needed.

Here is how I chose to setup my device/system, the target area(s) and purpose:

Device/System: Hub – Coordinates device integration and information flow.

Device/System: DVR/NVR – Stores image and video data for review, analysis and sharing.

Device/System: Internet – Facilitates remote sharing of information and interface with Hub.

Device/System: Smart Bulbs – Regulates lighting control (on, off, intensity).

Device/System: Cameras – Motion activation to capture activities at all doors (inside and outside), stairs, rooms (living and dining rooms, bedrooms, kitchen, basement, back porch), laundry area and HVAC area. Non motion activated focused on front and back yards.

Device/System: Motion Sensor – Helps trigger camera recording of camera-equipped rooms; detection of activity in non-camera equipped rooms, such as bathrooms.

Device/System: Open Sensor – Detects patterns of opening and closing of doors (front, back, refrigerator, cleaning cabinet).

Device/System: Temp Sensors – Detects the room temperature to adjust HVAC settings and alert to possible fire threats or threat of extreme cold.

Device/System: Water Sensor – Detects and prevents extensive damage from water on the floor.

Device/System: Smart Outlets – Controls on and off activity of plugged in items, such as lights, TV, stove.

Device/System: Smart Switches – Controls ceiling lights, fans, door lock releases and garage doors.

Device/System: Smart Thermostat – Detects and control the house temperature.

Device/System: Smart Valves – Controls energy flow, i.e. gas to stove and water supply to overflowing sinks or tub.

_Insight 33__: I was the best person to coordinate needed responses and no monitored program would have the background nor emotional investment to provide my level of care._

TECHNOLOGY SETUP LESSONS LEARNED

Balancing the need to know and the respect for privacy.

These are the things I learned through trying to create a safer living space for a curious, determined, and defiant mother who was suffering from dementia. All the technology and automation and best wishes will not work unless you learn and apply these lessons. Something in my mother's mind caused her to turn things off by unplugging them from the outlets. Consequently, she unplugged the automation hub, cameras and telephone.

Technology sometimes creates challenges for emotional and ethical needs. Cameras provide a form of invasion (revealing) into the areas they monitor. I deployed no bathroom cameras. I, at no time, needed nor wanted to see my mother in a state of undress. However, there is that risk if she decides to move about the house in her birthday suit.

All the technology, automation and best wishes will not work unless you learn and apply, at a minimum, these lessons. Just about all of the products and devices you will use require electrical power. The risk is loss of ability when the power goes out. Think about a life-support oxygen system and what happens when the power goes out. I highly recommend selecting hubs and devices that have a battery backup component.

Consider getting an uninterrupted power supply (Ups) / battery and plug in the hub and internet devices.

What most likely will not work when the electricity goes out:

- Cameras-without battery backup.

- Lighting - lamps, ceiling, and outside.

- Garage door openers - unless they have a battery backup.

- Stove ignitor-however the gas may still work.

- Refrigerator-make sure it stays closed.

What will work when the electricity goes out:

- Smoke detectors - they are battery backed-up.

- Door locks - they are battery operated.

- Motion sensors - they are battery operated.

- Hub - will send and receive signals and send texts.

The following suggestions help to create a stable and effective system for our needs. I highly recommend you consider doing the following or you are just throwing your technology system money out the window:

Device/System: Hub

Consideration: Password protect your hub. Lock the hub away in a cabinet to prevent tampering. Locate it in front of an outlet if possible.

Device/System: DVR/NVR

Consideration: Get enough storage to handle recording of all the cameras (I had twelve) for about 6 months: I suggest 3 terra bytes. Review and delete low value recordings or the recordings will get overwritten.

Device/System: Internet

Consideration: You need upload speed. That is what will send the videos and alerts to you. Get signal repeaters because some homes have dead spots. Consider placing one on each level, garage, and porch. Station the internet box out-of-reach of your loved one's hands and preferably sight.

Device/System: Smart Bulbs

Consideration: You can program these and activate with motion sensors. This helps illuminate rooms when your loved one enters at night. If the alert says they are offline, check the camera recordings to see if they have been removed or unplugged by your loved one.

Device/System: Cameras

Consideration: Position all cameras up high and out of reach. I choose the ceiling. You should install outlets in the areas of the camera (ceiling or high wall). My mother liked unplugging everything.

Device/System: Motion Sensor

Consideration: Get the kind that can double as a temperature sensor—this saves you money. I choose to get motion sensors to cover window areas. These usually have a field of view of 150 to 180 degrees, eliminating the need for open/close sensors for each window. Position them on stairways, in bathrooms, bedrooms, by the doors and anywhere you want to be alerted if someone goes into the respective area.

Device/System: Open Sensor

Consideration: Place these high up on doors or they will disappear. There are embedded door sensors, but you will need to drill holes in the door and frame.

Device/System: Temperature Sensors

Consideration: Use these to learn where it is hot or cold throughout the house. I also used two near the stove to sense a burner was left on and to trigger the Smart Valve (gas shut-off).

Device/System: Water Sensor

Consideration: These tend to go on the floor. Place them near sinks and toilets preferably out of sight or they will disappear. This came from having a bathroom sink overflow to the floor, to the first floor (ceiling, wall, floor), and to the basement (ceiling, wall and floor).

Device/System: Smart Outlets

Consideration: Just make sure you place locked covers on low-level ones or things get unplugged.

Device/System: Smart Thermostat

Consideration: Place a lock cover on this. My mom took it out of the wall twice.

Device/System: Smart Valves

Consideration: These will require professional installation and possible inspection and approval. Check with your installers. These can save lives. They saved us from catastrophic damage.

Device/System: Coded Door Locks

Consideration: You get an emergency set of keys, keep one on the property. You assign a code to each vital user. Setup a separate code for contractors needing repeat visits. Setup a one-time code (it is deleted after one usage) for emergency personnel (such as police, fire, neighbors). Use the code activity log (who's code was entered) along with the camera log to determine if there is a misuse (using someone else code) of the assigned codes. Battery replacement depends on frequency of usage.

Insight 34: *Have the electrician install outlets high on the wall or ceiling.*

Insight #35: *Have a backup because the primary systems can fail.*

Reginald A. Lawson

MANAGING THE SCENARIOS

Reginald A. Lawson

STRATEGIES AND TACTICS

Applying Understanding, Technology and Dementia Sense

The following scenarios are what you likely will encounter through the various dementia stages. The accompanying suggestions are what I found to be effective and efficient.

Here are my definitions for the terms used in this section:

- Focus – An area you most likely (from my direct and indirect experiences) will encounter and want to address.

- Scenario – An actual event I encountered under a specific focus.

- Need-To-Know – Key people this awareness would help in their understanding and decision-making regarding your loved one.

- Tool – The device(s) and or system(s) I used to address the scenario.

- Purpose – The intended help (detection, decision, action) to be gained from using the tool.

- Application – My approach using the respective tool.

- Staging – A common period where this may occur in the 7-stages of dementia.

- Considerations – Things to think about in the selection and placement of the tool; suggestions on how to turn data into useful information.

Remember, I was not living with my mother and it takes me at least two-hours to respond to a threat. Therefore, the smartest thing I could do was to gather accurate data and provide to others that could respond sooner.

Most automation products and systems are not designed to support dementia care. I had to re-purpose the parameters, placement, and usage of things to make them work for my needs.

Focus: Door Lock Status

- Scenario: Are the doors closed and/or locked?

- Need-To-Know: Caregiver, 1st responders.

- Tool: Open and close sensor, automated lock, camera.

- Purpose: To alert you of a need to secure the doors.

- Application: Place the sensors with one on the door and one on the frame.

- Staging: Use these beginning with stage three.

- Considerations: Recommend using coded automated locks on front and back doors. Keys get lost or hidden, stolen or duplicated. Some automated locks can be remotely locked/unlocked. Get software that provides a log of activity. The logs give you a baseline and quickly shows a change of pattern. Set alert for each time the door is in unlock mode.

Focus: Egress – exiting the house

- Scenario: Did they go out, did they leave the property, and in which direction, and when?

- Need-To-Know: Caregiver and first responders (if your loved one walks off).

- Tool: Exterior camera (or interior camera facing outside).

- Purpose: To determine (1) if they are in the outside area (front/back/side); (2) if they tend to, or actually, leave the property; (3) what they were wearing at the time they left; (4) what times they tend to go outside/left; and which direction they headed.

- Application: Place the camera to see the widest angle possible covering the walkway they would most likely use.

- Staging: Definitely at stage three—they start to forget their address and sometimes their name in this stage.

- Considerations: Recommend getting a camera system that provides a dvr/nvr to record activity. Reviewing the recording to detect their pattern(s) for going out (times and frequency), how far they tend to go, whether they seem confident or lost (looking uncertain and anxious), you may get to see how they interact with others.

Focus: Ingress – entering the house

- Scenario: Did they come back in, who else came in the house, when?

- Need-To-Know: Caregiver, first responders.

- Tool: Camera, open/close sensor.

- Purpose: To capture who comes into the home, what times and to determine threats.

- Application: Place the sensors on all external doors; place a camera to capture the door activity.

- Staging: Stage two, mainly because they may start not remembering who came in the house.

- Considerations: Place a camera to capture door activity, focus it so you can see a face clearly, get the type with motion detection. Set it to trigger when the open sensor detects opening, and to save pre-open activity (10 seconds before) and record for 1 to 1 1/2 minutes.

Focus: Bowel Movement /Bathroom Usage Frequency

- Scenario: Do they have regular bowel movements.

- Need-To-Know: Medical Team/ER Team.

- Tool: Motion sensor.

- Purpose: To detect and evaluate patterns of usage

- Application: Place the sensor to capture actual toilet usage only.

- Staging: Stage two.

- Considerations: This can be tricky. Set a motion sensor to only detects sitting on the toilet (this reduces sensing shower or hand washing activity) and be mindful they may try to remove the sensor. If that happens, set a sensor to capture when there is bathroom motion, then review the time spacing from alerts. You will be able to tell time spent on hand washing, having a bowel movement, showering and cleaning activities. FYI: **Toilet paper consumption is not a good indicator** as your loved one may use it for other things such as cleaning up or drying their hands.

Focus: Sleeping Patterns

- Scenario: Are they getting more or less sleep and when do they sleep?

- Need-To-Know: Caregiver, Medical Team.

- Tool: Camera, sensor.

- Purpose: To detect time and length of resting activity.

- Application: Place the camera to show the bed/resting area.

- Staging: Stage four.

- Considerations: Set the camera to motion detection. They will spend longer periods at rest as they progress through stages. Review the recordings to detect when and how long they tend to lie down, and how restful they are. They may sleep in different beds if they have the choice (a daytime bed, or a nighttime bed and in a room that is not cold).

Focus: Smoke/Carbon Monoxide/Fire Detection

- Scenario: Was there an occurrence of smoke, carbon monoxide or fire?

- Need-To-Know: Caregiver, first responders.

- Tool: Smoke detectors.

- Purpose: To detect alert types and frequency.

- Application: Place a detector on each level, and in enclosed patios, garages.

- Staging: Stage two.

- Considerations: I prefer the combo detectors, with voice announcements, lighting and wi-fi signaling. Make sure your devices link to your hub to allow notification and automated sequencing with other devices (fans, locks, windows, lighting). Review activity log for patterns to make possible adjustments in placement.

Focus: Pain Impacting Movement

- Scenario: They walk with a limp from pain on one side or in one leg.

- Need-To-Know: Caregiver, Medical Team, first responders.

- Tool: Camera.

- Purpose: To detect walking movement or balance issues.

- Application: Place cameras to capture movement in living room to kitchen.

- Staging: Stage three.

- Considerations: Set the camera view to observe at least seven steps. Check the recordings for early morning walking and after they have been sitting for a while either in living room or kitchen.

Focus: Lost Ability to Stand

- Scenario: Are they struggling to get up from a seated position or fall?

- Need-To-Know: Caregiver, Medical Team, 1st responders.

- Tool: Camera.

- Purpose: Capture movement control when lowering to sit or rising from sitting.

- Application: Place camera to capture seated areas (i.e. living room, dining room, kitchen).

- Staging: Stage three.

- Considerations: Soft seating (especially couches) requires more muscle strength and coordination to rise from because ii provides less support than a chair arm. It will be clear when rising effort becomes more challenging. Increase log reviews as they progress in stages.

Focus: Eating Pattern

- Scenario: Did they eat, and if so, when, what, where?

- Need-To-Know: Caregiver, Medical Team.

- Tool: Camera, sensor.

- Purpose: To detect eating time, place, type of food and amount consumed.

- Application: Focus camera on eating area, place sensor in food area.

- Staging: Stage three.

- Considerations: The timing, frequency, amount and comfort associated with eating will change. They can go from eating as soon as they wake to not eating at all. Their preferred types of food may change (they may go from solid-to-soft-to-liquid). They may prefer eating alone as they progress. Leave the food out and check later to see if it is in the trash.

Focus: Negotiating the Stairs

- Scenario: Are they having trouble going up/downstairs?

- Need-To-Know: Caregiver, Medical Team.

- Tool: Camera.

- Purpose: To detect how, and if, they negotiated the stairs.

- Application: Place to scan the entire staircase—use two if needed.

- Staging: Stage three.

- Considerations: Review the camera often. Your loved one may lean heavily to one side, or pause ascending or descending, or attempt to go then turn around; or they may completely depend on the handrail.

Focus: Fallen on Stairs

- Scenario: Have they fallen on the stairs?

- Need-To-Know: Caregiver, Medical Team, first responders.

- Tool: Camera.

- Purpose: To detect a fall.

- Application: Place camera(s) to view the entire staircase.

- Staging: Stage three.

- Considerations: Set camera to constantly record the stairs. Review the recording every day.

Focus: Independent Living

- Scenario: Can they still do laundry, wash dishes?

- Need-To-Know: Caregiver.

- Tool: Camera.

- Purpose: Detect forgetfulness, strength, mobility, decision-making.

- Application: Place camera to view washing area; set to record on motion.

- Staging: Stage three.

- Considerations: Review the recording to look for any sign of delay in selecting garments; signs of putting the wrong item in the washer/dryer (i.e. overcoat, book, detergent bottle); signs of turning washer on and walking away without loading; signs of using the incorrect cleaning agents (for dishes).

Focus: Attempted Wandering

- Scenario: They are attempting to leave the house.

- Need-To-Know: Caregiver.

- Tool: Sensor, camera, phone.

- Purpose: Detect and prevent leaving the house.

- Application: Place camera to view doors; pace sensor to capture motion near door.

- Staging: Stage three.

- Considerations: Place a camera to view the entire door; place a motion sensor to capture movement within five feet of the door; set the hub to alert you when motion is detected near the door. You can set up time periods to deactivate the sensor when others are with your loved one. My signal that my mother was leaving was her attire. She always put on a dress when she planned to attend an imaginary funeral. Once I saw her in a dress, I called her on the phone, inquired about her intentions and talked her out of it.

Focus: Kitchen stove burner status

- Scenario: Are the kitchen burners on?

- Need-To-Know: Caregivers.

- Tool: Camera, temperature sensors, gas shut-off valve or electrical outlet.

- Purpose: To immediately detect and prevent this life-threatening event.

- Application: Place a camera to see the entire stove, place a heat sensor above the stove and set alert to a heat higher than normal cooking; install an automatic gas shutoff valve or plug stove into a controllable outlet.

- Staging: Stage Three.

- Considerations: Recommend having the cameras record stove activity at all times, then review the recording to detect when and how often they use the stove. Once you see they have left the burner on the first time, then do two things 1) set the stove to be able to come on only at certain times, then to turn off; 2) set the stove to be turned off by the stove heat sensor when it detect higher than normal stove heat. Have the system alert you immediately each time.

MY HOPE FOR YOU

Appreciate the progress you will make.

I know this book does not cover all the challenges you may face. I know at-home stay does not fit everyone's situation. I believe there are things involved in saying at home that have immeasurable value. Adjust your approaches to what you, your loved one and the circumstances can tolerate.

It is in that spirit that I have provided this book. You now have the benefit of my experiences. My prayer is that something within these pages is useful to you and sustains you through this time of challenges and revelations.

Go beyond this book; seek the comfort, experiences and wisdom of others who are taking this long walk, too. In sharing your experiences, you will find support and strength. I close by saluting your efforts to provide a safer at-home stay for your loved one. It is not an easy effort, and it is certainly not for everyone or every situation.

I sincerely hope this information positions you to have many successes early and often—successes that give you peace and solace in your journey.

REFERENCES

Give Your Parents A Standing Ovation! – For Caregivers of
Elderly Parents
Dr. Gybrilla Ballard-Blakes

10 Things a Person Living with Dementia Would Tell You If
They Could
Bob DeMarco at 2/26/2018 12:05 p.m.

The Amazing Village in The Netherlands Just for People with
Dementia
https://twistedsifter.com/2015/02/amazing-village-in-
netherlands-just-for-people-with-dementia/

Boost your brain power with the right nutrition
Liz Weinandy, RD Nov 14, 2018 Healthy Eating Cognitive and
Memory Disorders

6 Reasons Why You Might Have to Put Someone with
Dementia in a Memory Care Facility or Nursing Home
Bob DeMarco Alzheimer's Reading Room

The Mini-Cog Test for Alzheimer's and Dementia
Bob DeMarco Alzheimer's Reading Room

ACKNOWLEDGEMENTS

First, I thank GOD for my mother. I thank my mother for her love, teachings, strength and role-modeling of courage.

I want to acknowledge my sister Vicky, cousins George and Elyse, and Ms. Shirley for their unselfish, direct and timely stepping in to help. I want to acknowledge the service providers and involved friends who were gifts to us and made seemingly impossible solutions workable:

- *Dr. Debrah Zarek and Dr. Ina Li and their staff for their knowledge and compassion.*

- *Attorney James Owens for his guidance and care taking style.*

- *Kimberly Carson, our paid caregiver and beacon for showing us how to be steady on the journey.*

- *Byron and Brandon Milam, our trusted general contractors, for their gifted spirits and assistance in getting things working.*

- *Ron Seeney, our electrician for adding lights and enlightenment.*

- *Gayle Mabrey, RN, Seasons Hospice Care for her positive demeanor.*

- *Joye Mercer Barksdale, for reading and editing my manuscript and providing rich encouraging perspectives to guide this effort.*

- *Sherrin Ingram, for her spirit of giving and helping me overcome the final hurdles to reach my launch goal.*

- *Scott Allan, my SPS writing, launch, and marketing coach for his guidance and examples of success.*

- *Dr. Flavia Walton and her incredible team of caregivers at Dementia Friendly America, Prince Georg's County South for continued enhancement of my understanding about dementia.*

- *Shaunda Bellamy, President, Pickett Fences Senior Services Inc, for her encouraging support of my efforts to help others.*

Lastly and most importantly, I acknowledge my loved ones, friends and mother's neighbors for their understanding and support through my years of caring for my mother.

ABOUT THE AUTHOR

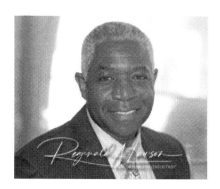

Reginald A. Lawson has been helping people most of his life. He is a son, brother, father, friend and mostly decent neighbor. His background includes law enforcement, computer programming, volunteering at food banks, coaching and officiating kids' sports, serving as an HOA President, CEO of his own company, and coaching and training leaders.

Knowing how to listen, assess, evaluate, make decisions, test and implement solutions, and critique results are part of his pre-caregiving skillset.

His post caregiving skillset includes how to hear the look in a needing eye, distinguish the cry for help inside anger, understand deeper the power of silence and touch, and how to turn off intellect and live through a greater spirit. He is more humbled, honored, enlighten, thankful and at peace.

Reginald A. Lawson is available for speaking engagements, and design consultation for dementia caregiving automation systems. Send request to info@sbgpc.com.

Reginald A. Lawson lives in Maryland, United States.

You can connect with Reginald online at:
www.sbgpc.com/caregivers or ralawson@sbgpc.com

ENDNOTES

[1] Dementia Patients Can Deceive Others to the Distress of Their Caregiver
Bob DeMarco, Alzheimer's Reading Room, Mar 22, 2018

[2] Non-Alzheimer's Causes of Dementia – How to tell the difference
Paula Spencer Scott, Senior Health Writer

[3] What is the Difference Between Alzheimer's and Dementia
Bob DeMarco, Alzheimer's Reading Room, Nov 20, 2018

[4] Dementia Care Central – Stages of Alzheimer's & Dementia: Durations & Scales Used to Measure Progression: GDS, FAST & CDR, Sep 1, 2018

[5] Revocable vs. Irrevocable Living Trust
Julie Garber, www.thebalance.com

[6] When A Person Living With Dementia Gets Angry and Confused
Bob DeMarco, Alzheimer's Reading Room

[7] Alzheimer's: Tips to make holidays more enjoyable
https://www.mayoclinic.org/healthy-lifestyle/caregivers/in-depth/alzheimers/art-20047715

Made in the USA
Middletown, DE
23 June 2023

33331794R00087